Book 1

MRCP

Practice Questions & Answers

Cardiology and Respiratory Medicine

Edited by

Philip Kelly MBBS MRCP
Department of Diabetes and Metabolism
Royal London Hospital
London

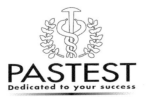

PASTEST
Dedicated to your success

© 2005 PASTEST Ltd
Egerton Court
Parkgate Estate
Knutsford
Cheshire
WA16 8DX

Telephone: 01565 752000

First published 2005

ISBN: 1 904627 25 0

A catalogue record for this book is available from the British Library.

The information contained within this book was obtained by the authors from reliable sources. However, while every effort has been made to ensure its accuracy, no responsibility for loss, damage or injury occasioned to any person acting or refraining from action as a result of information contained herein can be accepted by the publishers or authors.

PasTest Revision Books and Intensive Courses

PasTest has been established in the field of postgraduate medical education since 1972, providing revision books and intensive study courses for doctors preparing for their professional examinations. Books and courses are available for the following specialties:

MRCGP, MRCP Part 1 and 2, MRCPCH Part 1 and 2, MRCPsych, MRCS, MRCOG, DRCOG, DCH, FRCA, PLAB.

For further details contact:

PasTest, Freepost, Knutsford, Cheshire WA16 7BR
Tel: 01565 752000 Fax: 01565 650264
www.pastest.co.uk enquiries@pastest.co.uk

Text prepared by Vision Typesetting Ltd, Manchester
Printed and bound by Cambrian Printers, Aberystwyth

CONTENTS

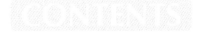

Cardiology
James Wilkinson MRCP(UK) MB BS BSc(Hons)
British Heart Foundation Research Fellow and Specialist Registrar in Cardiology, Wolfson Institute for Biomedical Research, University College London, London.

Respiratory Medicine
Susannah Leaver MBBS BmedSci(Hons) MRCP(UK)
Specialist Registrar in Respiratory Medicine, South West Thames Rotation.

ACKNOWLEDGEMENTS

I would like to express my gratitude to the team at PasTest, particularly Cathy Dickens and Amy Smith for their unswerving support and tolerance during the preparation of this series. Many patients have been gracious enough to contribute to our ongoing education by allowing their images to be used in these volumes. The series would have been impossible without the help of the following: Dr A Jain, Specialist Registrar, Cardiology, The London Chest Hospital; Dr P McCoubrie, Consultant Radiologist, Bristol; Dr Y Ho, Bromptom Hospital; Dr E Behr, Cardiology Specialist Registrar, St. George's Hospital; Dr N Hughes, Consultant Radiologist, Frimley Park Hospital; Dr R Knight, Consultant Respiratory Physician, Frimley Park Hospital; Dr Michael Ardern-Jones, Specialist Registrar Dermatology, Oxford Radcliffe NHS Trust; Dr Tim Ho, Consultant Respiratory Physician, Frimley Park Hospital and Dr Heather Jefferson, Specialist Registrar in Nephrology for proofreading the respiratory section.

Philip Kelly

The MRCP (UK) Part 2 written examination consists of two 3-hour papers, each with up to 100 multiple choice questions; they are either one from five (best of 5) or 'n' from many, where two answers are chosen from ten. Each question will have a clinical scenario and might contain investigations to interpret; many might also contain an image. There is a pass-mark agreed by the examiners but a candidate's performance is also assessed in relation to other candidates.

This three book series provides practice questions with extensive explanations to aid candidates preparing for the examination. The authors are all clinicians writing sections in their chosen fields and as such have been chosen for their clear understanding of the required knowledge base for this important exam. The breadth of knowledge for this exam is vast and they have attempted to cover the 'syllabus' as completely as possible. Great care has been taken to explain areas that cause difficulty as thoroughly as possible. No apology is made where the format of the questions differs slightly from the exam. These books are not merely practice papers but educational aids and where a topic can be best explained by diversion from the strict format of the exam, for the sake of understanding, this has been done.

This book covers cardiology and respiratory medicine and is best taken – in concert with its colleagues within the series – as a supplement to a thorough clinical grounding, the general medical texts and the core clinical journals.

Any comments or suggestions on this book or the series will be gratefully received.

Haematology

Full blood count

Haemoglobin (Hb):	
males	13.0–18.0 g/dL
females	11.5–16.5 g/dL
Haematocrit (Hct/PCV):	
males	0.40–0.52
females	0.36–0.47
Mean corpuscular volume (MCV)	80–96 fL
Mean corpuscular Hb(MCH)	28–32 pg
Mean corpuscular Hb concentration (MCHC)	32–35 g/dL
White cell count (WCC)	$4–11 \times 10^9$/L
DifferentialWCC:	
Neutrophils	$1.5–7 \times 10^9$/L
Lymphocytes	$1.5–4 \times 10^9$/L
Monocytes	$0–0.8 \times 10^9$/L
Eosinophils	$0.04–0.4 \times 10^9$/L
Basophils	$0–0.1 \times 10^9$/L
Platetlets	$150–400 \times 10^9$/L
Reticulocytes	$25–85 \times 10^9$/L
Erythrocyte sedimentation rate (ESR):	
Under 50 years	
males	0–15 mm/h
females	0–20 mm/h
Over 50 years	
males	0–20 mm/h
females	0–30 mm/h

Coagulation

Prothrombin time (PT)	11.5–15.5 s
International normalised ratio (INR)	< 1.4

Activated partial thromboplastin time (APTP)   30–40 s
Fibrinogen   1.8–5.4 g/L
Bleeding time   3–8 min

Coagulation factors

Factors II, V, VII, VIII, IX, X, XI, XII   50–150 U/dL
von Willebrand factor   45–150 U/dL
Protein C   80–135 U/dL
Protein S   80–120 U/dL
Fibrin degradation products (FDP)   <100 mg/L
D-Dimer screen   < 0.5 mg/L

Haematinics

Serum iron   12–30 µmol/L
Serum total iron-binding capacity (TIBC)   45–75 µmol/L
Serum ferritin   15–300 µg/L
Serum B_{12} 160–760 ng/L
Serum folate   2.0–11.0 µg/L
Red cell folate   160–640 µg/L
Haemoglobin electrophoresis:
  Haemoglobin A   >95%
  Haemoglobin A_2 2–3%
  Haemoglobin F   < 2%

Chemistry

Sodium   137–144 mmol/L
Potassium   3.5–4.9 mmol/L
Chloride   95–107 mmol/L
Bicarbonate   20–28 mmol/L
Anion gap   12–16 mmol/L
Urea   2.5–7.5 mmol/L
Creatinine   60–110 µmol/L
Corrected calcium   2.2–2.6 mmol/L
Phosphate   0.8–1.4 mmol/L

Total protein   61–76 g/L
Albumin   37–49 g/L
Total bilirubin   1–22 µmol/L
Conjugated bilirubin   0–3.4 µmol/L
Alanine aminotransferase (ALT)   5–35 U/L
Aspartate aminotransferase (AST)   1–31 U/L
Alkaline phosphatase (ALP)   45–105 U/L(> 14 y)
Gamma glutamyl transferase (γGT)   4–35 U/L (< 50 in ♂)
Lactate dehydrogenase (LDH)   10–250 U/L

Creatine kinase (CK)	24–170 U/L (< 190 ♂)
Copper	12–26 µmol/L
Caeruloplasmin	200–350 mg/L
Magnesium	0.75–1.05 mmol/L
Urate (uric acid):	
males	0.23–0.46 mmol/L
females	0.19–0.36 mmol/L
Serum angiotensin-converting enzyme (ACE)	25–82 U/L
Fasting plasma glucose	3.0–6.0 mmol/L
Hb A_{1C}	3.8–6.4%
Serum amylase	60–180 U/L
Plasma osmolality	278–305 mosmol/kg

Lipids and lipoproteins

(targets vary, depending on cardiovascular risk)

Cholesterol	< 5.2 mmol/L
LDL cholesterol	< 3.36 mmol/L
HDL cholesterol	> 1.55 mmol/L
Fasting triglyceride	0.45–1.69 mmol/L

Blood gases (sea level, breathing air)

pH	7.36–7.44
P_{O_2}	11.3–12.6 kPa
P_{CO_2}	4.7–6.0 kPa
Base excess	± 2 mmol/L

Endocrinology

Adrenal steroids
Blood

Cortisol:	
09.00 h	200–700 nmol/L
22.00 h	5–250 nmol/L
Dehydroepiandrosterone sulphate (DHEAS):	
males	2–10 µmol/L
females	3–12 µmol/L
Plasma angiotensin II	5–35 pmol/L
Plasma renin activity:	
recumbent	1.1–2.7 pmol/ml/h
erect after 30 min	3.0–4.3 pmol/ml/h

Urine

Aldosterone	14–53 nmol/24h
Cortisol	55–250 nmol/24h

Pancreatic and gut hormones

Plasma gastrin	< 55 pmol/L
Plasma or serum insulin:	
overnight fasting	< 186 pmol/L
after hypoglycaemia	< 21 pmol/L
(blood glucose < 2.2 mmol/L)	
Plasma vasoactive intestinal peptide (VIP)	< 30 pmol/L
Plasma pancreatic polypeptide	< 300 pmol/L
Plasma glucagon	< 50 pmol/L

Thyroid hormones

Plasma thyroid-binding globulin	13–28 mg/L
Plasma thyroxine (T_4)	58–174 nmol/L
Free T_4	10–22 pmol/L
Thyroid stimulating hormone (TSH)	0.4–5 mU/L

Others

Plasma parathyroid hormone	0.9–5.4 pmol/L
Plasma calcitonin	< 27 pmol/L
Plasma antidiuretic hormone	0.9–4.6 pmol/L

Immunology/Rheumatolology

C-reactive protein (CPR)	< 10 mg/L
Serum immunoglobulins:	
IgG	6.0–13.0 g/L
IgA	0.8–3.0 g/L
IgM	0.4–2.5 g/L
IgE	< 120 kU/L
β_2-Microglobulin	< 3 mg/L
Antinuclear antibodies	negative at 1:20
Anti-dsDNA (ELISA)	0–73 U/ml
Rheumatoid factor	< 30 kU/L

Tumour markers

α-Fetoprotein (AFP)	< 10 kU/L (< 10 ng/ml)
Carcinoembryonic antigen (CEA)	< 10 µg/L (< 3 ng/ml)
Prostate-specific antigen (PSA):	
males over 40	< 4 µg/L
males under 40	< 2 µg/L
Human chorionic gonadotrophin (HCG)	< 5 U/L
CA 125	< 35 U/ml
CA 19-9	< 33 U/ml

Therapeutic drug levels

Plasma carbamazepine	34–51 µmol/L
Plasma digoxin (at least 6 h post-dose)	1–2 nmol/L
Blood gentamicin (peak)	5–7 µg/ml
Serum lithium	0.5–1.5 mmol/L
Serum phenobarbital	65–172 µmol/L
Serum phenytoin	40–80 µmol/L

Cerebrospinal fluid

Opening pressure	50–180 mmH$_2$O
Total protein	0.15–0.45 g/L
Albumin	0.066–0.442 g/L
Glucose	3.3–4.4 mmol/L
Cell count	⩽5/ml
Differential cell count:	
Lymphocytes	60–70%
Monocytes	30–50%
Neutrophils	none

Urine

Glomerular filtration rate (GFR)	70–140 ml/min
Total protein	< 0.2 g/24 h
Albumin	< 30 mg/24 h
5-hydroxyindoleacetic acid (5-HIAA)	10–47 µmol/24 h
Osmolality	350–1000 mosmol/kg
Albumin/creatinine ratio (untimed specimen):	
males	< 2.5 mg/mmol
females	< 3.5 mg/mmol

A&E	Accident and Emergency (Department)
Ab	Antibody
ABPA	Allergic bronchopulmonary aspergillosis
ACE	Angiotensin-converting enzyme
ADH	Antidiuretic hormone
AF	Atrial fibrillation
Ag	Antigen
AICD	Automatic implantable cardioverter/defibrillator
AIHA	Autoimmune haemolytic anaemia
ALL	Acute lymphoblastic leukaemia
ALP	Alkaline phosphatase
ALT	Alanine aminotranferase
AML	Acute myeloblastic (/myelocytic/myeloid) leukaemia
ANA	Antinuclear antibody
ANCA	Anti-neutrophil cytoplasmic antibody
Anti-Ach R	Anti-acetylcholine receptor
APKD	Adult polycystic kidney disease
APS	Antiphospholipid syndrome
APTT	Activated partial thromboplastin time
ARF	Acute renal failure
ASD	Atrial septal defect
ASOT	Antistreptolysin-O titre
AST	Aspartate aminotransferase
ATLL	Adult T-cell leukaemia/lymphoma
ATN	Acute tubular necrosis
BAL	Bronchoalveolar lavage
BMD	Bone mineral density
BMI	Body mass index
BTS	British Thoracic Society
CAH	Chronic active hepatitis
CAPD	Continuous ambulatory peritoneal dialysis
CCU	Coronary Care Unit

CHOP	Cyclophosphamide, doxorubicin hydrochloride, vincristine (Oncovin®), prednisolone (chemotherapy)
CJD	Creutzfeld–Jakob disease
CK	Creatine kinase
CLL	Chronic lymphoblastic leukaemia/chronic lymphocytic leukaemia
CMV	Cytomegalovirus
CNS	Central nervous system
CO_2	Carbon dioxide
COPD	Chronic obstructive pulmonary disease
CPAP	Continuous positive airway pressure (ventilation)
CPR	Cardiopulmonary resuscitation
CRF	Chronic renal failure
CRP	C-reactive protein
CRPA	Complex regional pain syndrome
CSF	Cerebrospinal fluid
CT	Computed tomography
CXR	Chest X-ray
DCT	Direct Coombs' test
DEXA	Dual-energy X-ray absorptiometry
DHES	Dehydroepiandrosterone sulphate
DIC	Disseminated intravascular coagulation
DIP	Distal interphalangeal (joint)
DKA	Diabetic ketoacidosis
DM	Diabetes mellitus
DMARD	Disease-modifying antirheumatic drug
DVT	Deep vein thrombosis
EBV	Epstein–Barr virus
ECG	Electrocardiogram
ECT	Electroconvulsive therapy
EEG	Electroencephalogram
ELISA	Enzyme-linked immunosorbent assay
EMG	Electromyogram
ENA	Extractable antinuclear antibody
ERCP	Endoscopic retrograde cholangiopancreatography
ESR	Erythrocyte sedimentation rate
ESRF	End-stage renal failure
FAP	Familial adenomatous poyposis
FEV_1	Forced expiratory volume in 1 second
FFP	Fresh frozen plasma
FMF	Familial Mediterranean fever
FVC	Forced vital capacity
G6PD	Glucose 6-phospate dehydrogenase
GBM	Glomerular basement membrane

GCS	Glasgow Coma Scale
GFR	Glomerular filtration rate
GORD	Gastro-oesophageal reflux disease
GP	General practitioner
GTN	Glyceryl trinitrate
HAV	Hepatitis A virus
Hb	Haemoglobin
HBV	Hepatitis B virus
HCC	Hepatocellular carcinoma
HCV	Hepatitis C virus
HDG	Human chorionic gonadotrophin
HDL	High-density lipoprotein
HELLP	Haemolysis, elevated liver function tests, low platelets
HEV	Hepatitis E virus
HHT	Hereditary haemorrhagic telangiectasia
HIV	Human immunodeficiency virus
HLA	Human leucocyte antigen
HNPCC	Hereditary non-polyposis colorectal cancer
HONK	Hyperosmolar non-ketotic state
HS	Hereditary spherocytosis
HSP	Henoch–Schönlein purpura
HTLV-1	Human T-cell leukaemia virus 1
IBD	Inflammatory bowel disease
ICU/ITU	Intensive Care Unit/Intensive Therapy Unit
INR	International normalised ratio
IPD	Intermittent peritoneal dialysis
IPSID	Immunoproliferative small-intestinal disease
ITP	Immune thrombocytopaenia
IUGR	Intrauterine growth retardation
IVC	Inferior vena cava
IVP	Intravenous pyelography
IVU	Intravenous urography
JIA	Juvenile idiopathic arthritis
JVP	Jugular venous pulse/pressure
Kco	Transfer coefficient
LDH	Lactate dehydrogenase
LDL	Low-density lipoprotein
LFT	Liver function test
LOS	Lower oesophageal sphincter
LP	Lumbar puncture
MAHA	Microangiopathic haemolytic anaemia
MAOI	Monoamine oxidase inhibitor
MCGN	Mesangiocapillary glomerulonephritis
MCH	Mean corpuscular haemoglobin

MCHC	Mean corpuscular haemoglobin concentration
MCP	Metacarpophalangeal (joint)
MCU	Micturating cystourography
MCV	Mean corpuscular volume
MDMA	3,4-methylene dioxymethamphetamine (Ecstasy)
MEN	Multiple endocrine neoplasia
MI	Myocardial infarction
MIBG	Metaiodobenzylguanidine
MODS	Multiple-organ dysfunction syndrome
MPO	Myeloperoxidase
MRA	Magnetic resonance angiogram
MRI	Magnetic resonance imaging
MS	Multiple sclerosis
MSA	Multiple systems atrophy
MSU	Mid-stream urine (sample)
MTP	Metatarsophalangeal (joint)
NHL	Non-Hodgkin's lymphoma
NICE	National Institute for Clinical Excellence
NIV	Non-invasive ventilation
NSAID	Non-steroidal anti-inflammatory drug
O_2	Oxygen
OA	Ostroarthritis
PA	Pernicious anaemia/pulmonary artery
PAN	Polyarteritis nodosa
PBC	Primary biliary cirrhosis
PCOS	Polycystic ovary syndrome
PCP	*Pneumocystis carinii* pneumonia
PCR	Polymerase chain reaction
PCV	Packed cell volume
PDA	Patent ductus arteriosus
PE	Pulmonary embolus
PEF(R)	Peak expiratory flow (rate)
PFT	Pulmonary function test
PIP	Proximal interphalangeal (joint)
PMR	Polymyalgia rheumatica
PNH	Paroxysmal nocturnal haemoglobinuria
PSA	Prostate-specific antigen
PSC	Primary sclerosing cholangitis
PT	Prothrombin time
PTH	Parathyroid hormone
RA	Rheumatoid arthritis
RAST	radioallergosorbent test
RCC	Renal cell carcinoma
RCC/RBC	Red cell count/red blood cell

RDW	Red cell distribution width
REM	Rapic eye movement
RSD	Reflex sympathetic dystrophy
RSV	Respiratory syncytial virus
RTA	Renal tubular acidosis/road traffic accident
RV	Right ventricle/residual volume
RVOT	Right ventricular outflow tract
SCD	Sickle cell disease
SHBG	Sex hormone-binding globulin
SIADH	Syndrome of inappropriate ADH secretion
SLE	Systemic lupus erythematosus
SOD	Sphincter of Oddi dysfunction
Spo_2	Oxygen saturation, measured by pulse oximetry
SSRI	Serotonin reuptake inhibitor
SVT	Supraventricular tachycardia
TB	Tuberculosis
TCC	Transitional cell carcinoma
TIA	Transient ischaemic attack
TLC	Total lung capacity
T_{LCO}	Transfer factor of the lung for carbon monoxide (= D_{LCO})
TNF	Tumour necrosis factor
TOE	Transoesophageal echocardiogram
tPA	Tissue-type plasminogen activator
TPN	Total parenteral nutrition
TRUS	Transrectal ultrasound
TSH	Thyroid stimulating hormone
TT	Thrombin time
TTP	Thrombotic thrombocytopaenic purpura
U&Es	Urea and electrolytes
US	Ultrasound
UTI	Urinary tract infection
VF	Ventricular fibrillation
VSD	Ventricular septal defect
VT	Ventricular tachycardia
vWD	von Willebrand's disease
WCC/WBC	White cell count/white blood cell
WG	Wegener's granulomatosis
WPW	Wolff–Parkinson–White (syndrome)
γGT	Gamma glutamyltransferase

Chapter One

CARDIOLOGY

Case 1

A 38-year-old man presented to A&E with retrosternal chest pain, which he had had for 7 hours.

On examination he looked comfortable but was tachycardic and pyrexial; his physical examination was otherwise normal. His troponin T is mildly elevated. His ECG is shown below:

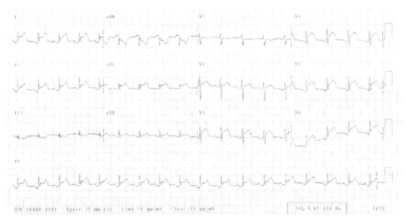

Image provided by Dr J Wilkinson, Cardiology Research Fellow, University College London, London

1   What is the most likely diagnosis?

- A   ST-elevation myocardial infarct
- B   Brugada syndrome
- C   Non-ST-elevation myocardial infarct
- D   Pericarditis
- E   Gastro-oesophageal reflux disease (GORD)

Case 2

You are referred a 45-year-old man with chest pain, which he describes as a dull epigastric/lower chest ache that came on when he ran for a bus, shortly after a large meal, and lasted about 20 minutes before easing off. He is obese and known to have GORD.

Physical examination is normal. His initial ECG shows some flattening of his T waves in the lateral leads but his most recent ECG is normal. The troponin T, taken 6 hours after the patient said the pain started, is normal.

1   Which of the following would be most appropriate?

- [ ] A   Reassure him, prescribe a proton pump inhibitor and discharge him to his GP
- [ ] B   Reassure him, prescribe him a GTN spray, discharge him and arrange for him to come back for an exercise test in 6 weeks
- [ ] C   Give him thrombolytic therapy and admit him to the Coronary Care Unit (CCU)
- [ ] D   Reassure him, discharge him and tell him to see his GP if he has any further symptoms
- [ ] E   Admit him, treat him as if he had acute coronary syndrome and repeat his troponin in 12 hours

Case 3

A 70-year-old lady has an out-of-hospital cardiac arrest; when the paramedics arrive on scene she is in VF. They successfully cardiovert her, resuscitate her on-scene and transfer her to A&E. On arrival she is stable and in sinus rhythm. The following day she is well and there is no evidence of an MI or of any other precipitating cause.

She had an inferior MI one year ago, for which she received thrombolysis. An angiogram, done privately 6 months ago, showed unobstructed coronaries with plaque disease, inferior hypokinesia and an ejection fraction of 30%. She is on ramipril, aspirin and a statin and has been asymptomatic with normal exercise tolerance.

1 Which of the following describes how she should be best managed?

- [ ] A Put on oral amiodarone and discharge
- [ ] B Do an exercise test and discharge if it is normal
- [ ] C Have an automatic implantable cardioverter defibrillator (AICD) inserted prior to discharge
- [ ] D Reassure and discharge
- [ ] E Put on a β-blocker and nitrate and discharge with an exercise test booked for 6 weeks' time

Case 4

A senior house officer presents their clerking of a young man they have seen in clinic, the patient presented with a 6-month history of worsening shortness of breath on exertion, occasional dizzy spells and blackouts.

On examination the senior house officer found the patient to have a loud ejection systolic murmur at the left sternal edge. The pulse and blood pressure were both normal and the remainder of the cardiovascular examination was normal. In the notes you notice there is a picture of the patient as a child (shown below). The senior house officer has requested an echo and has arranged for the patient to be seen as a follow up in two weeks with the results. The senior house officer asks you what the most likely diagnosis is, to put in their clinic letter to the GP.

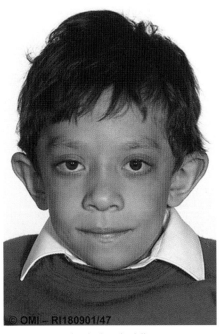

© OMI – RI180901/47

Image courtesy of Oxford Medical Illustration

1   Which statement most accurately describes the diagnosis?

☐ A Congenital bicuspid aortic valve, which is severely stenotic, with Turner's syndrome

☐ B Congenital bicuspid aortic valve, which is severely stenotic, with Noonan's syndrome

☐ C Hypertrophic cardiomyopathy and DiGeorge syndrome

☐ D Pulmonary stenosis and Noonan's syndrome

☐ E Pulmonary stenosis and Turner's syndrome

Case 5

Below is the ECG from leads V1–3 (the ECG recording from all other leads, not shown, is normal) of a young man presenting with a history of blackouts. He is on no medication, takes no drugs or alcohol and has no family history of note. His physical examination is normal.

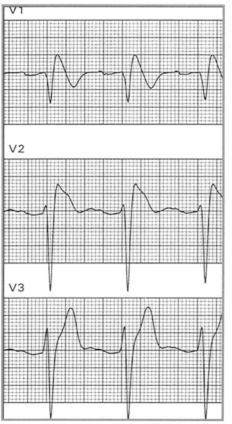

Image provided by Dr E Behr, Specialist Registrar in Cardiology, St George's Hospital, London

1   What is the diagnosis?

- ☐   A   Vasovagal syncope
- ☐   B   Brugada syndrome
- ☐   C   Hypertrophic cardiomyopathy
- ☐   D   Wolff–Parkinson–White syndrome
- ☐   E   Jervell and Lange-Nielsen syndrome

Case 6

The surgeons admitted an 18-year-old man with left iliac fossa pain. He had a history of recurrent sinusitis but no other medical problems.

On examination there were no murmurs, his blood pressure and pulse were normal and he had rebound tenderness and guarding in his left iliac fossa. Below is his chest X-ray:

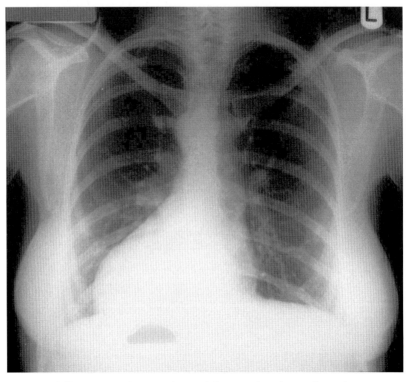

Image provided by Dr P McCoubrie, Consultant Radiologist, Southmead Hospital, Bristol

1   What does his chest X-ray show?

- ☐ A   Dextrocardia
- ☐ B   Free air under the diaphragm
- ☐ C   Situs inversus
- ☐ D   Kartagener's syndrome
- ☐ E   Situs solitus

Case 7

A 70-year-old man has a blackout and collapses without warning while playing bowls. By the time he reaches hospital he is fine. He has no past medical history, is on no drugs and has normal exercise tolerance.

On examination he looks well; there is an ejection systolic murmur with a quiet second heart sound. His pulse volume is reduced. There are no other signs. His ECG shows left bundle branch block and sinus rhythm. All his blood tests are normal.

1   Which of the following is the most appropriate next step?

- ☐   A   Ensure he has an inpatient echocardiogram prior to discharge
- ☐   B   Give him thrombolysis for his new anterior MI
- ☐   C   Arrange an exercise test
- ☐   D   Arrange an outpatient echo and follow-up
- ☐   E   Arrange an outpatient Holter test

Case 8

A 26-year-old patient is referred to you by A&E having collapsed; she has had increasing breathlessness and fatigue over the last week. Apart from a transient rash while she was away on holiday, which she put down to heat rash, she has no past medical history and is not on any medication. She takes no alcohol, tobacco or drugs. She is a very fit cross-country runner, having just returned from the World Championships in New England. Her previous medical and ECG 2 years ago were normal, as required by the Athletics Association.

She feels very unwell, dizzy and has difficulty standing; her blood pressure is 80/40 mmHg. Apart from this and a bradycardia, her examination is otherwise normal. Below is her ECG:

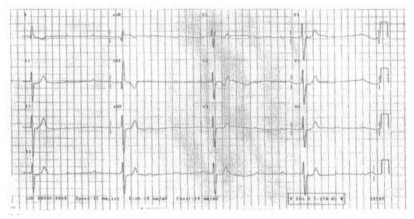

Image provided by Dr J Wilkinson, Cardiology Research Fellow, University College London, London

1   Which of the following describes how she should best be managed?

- ☐ A   Insertion of a dual-chamber pacemaker
- ☐ B   Medical therapy
- ☐ C   Do an invasive electrophysiological study with a view to definitive treatment
- ☐ D   Insertion of temporary pacing wire to allow further diagnostic tests and management
- ☐ E   Perform an angiogram to rule out a silent inferior MI

Case 9

A 23-year-old lady who is known to suffer from recurrent supraventricular tachycardia (SVT) presents with palpitations and an SVT.

She carries her resting ECG with her, which is shown below. Her recent echocardiogram was normal. She is not haemodynamically compromised and there is no evidence of pulmonary oedema. She has no other medical problems apart from asthma, for which she is on inhalers.

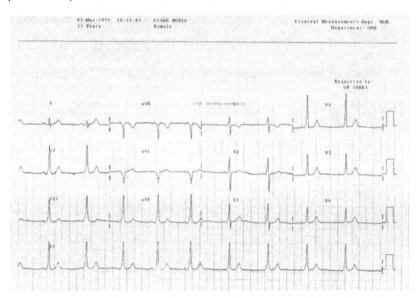

Image provided by Dr J Wilkinson, Cardiology Research Fellow, University College London, London

1 How should she best be managed?

- [ ] A Intravenous adenosine
- [ ] B DC cardioversion
- [ ] C Intravenous verapamil
- [ ] D Intravenous digoxin
- [ ] E Intravenous flecainide

Case 10

A 53-year-old man on the Coronary Care Unit (CCU) suddenly develops cardiogenic shock 5 days after his initial inferior ST-elevation MI, for which he received thrombolysis.

The salient features on examination are: pulse 120 bpm, BP 75/50 mmHg, pansystolic murmur, florid pulmonary oedema. A right heart catheter is inserted to help guide management and the following readings are noted:

Central venous saturation	55%
Pulmonary artery saturations	80%

1   Which of the following describes the diagnosis and best management (assume your clinical diagnosis has been confirmed with an urgent echo)?

☐   A   Ischaemic mitral regurgitation due to ruptured papillary muscle needing urgent intra-aortic balloon pump and referral for surgery

☐   B   Right ventricular rupture needing urgent surgery

☐   C   Ischaemic ventricular septal defect needing urgent intra-aortic balloon pump and referral for surgery

☐   D   Ischaemic ventricular septal defect needing medical therapy with inotropes

☐   E   Ischaemic ventricular septal defect needing urgent intra-aortic balloon pump and urgent interventional radiology

Case 11

At 2 o'clock in the morning a 72-year-old lady presents to the District General Hospital where you are on call. She has central crushing chest pain of 3 hours' duration and breathlessness. She has recently been diagnosed with diabetes mellitus (started on diet control) and smokes five cigarettes a day. She is otherwise fit, fully independent and is on no medical treatment.

Her ECG is shown below:

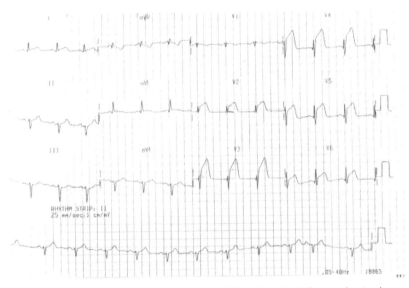

Image provided by Dr J Wilkinson, Cardiology Research Fellow, University College London, London

1 Which of the following is the most appropriate statement?

☐ A Put her on a heparin infusion while you call a cardiologist (who is on call from home) at your local intervention centre, which is more than 3 hours drive away, to discuss the possibility of angioplasty

☐ B Put her on a low molecular weight heparin, glycoprotein IIb/IIIa antagonist infusion and GTN infusion. Admit her to CCU and consider angiography the next day if her symptoms have not settled

☐ C Administer thrombolysis, provided there are no contraindications (streptokinase and intravenous heparin)

☐ D Administer thrombolysis, provided there are no contraindications (tPA and intravenous heparin) and start her on clopidogrel in addition to standard therapy

☐ E Administer thrombolysis, provided there are no contraindications (tPA and intravenous heparin)

Case 12

A 26-year-old lady presents with sudden-onset pulmonary oedema, for which she has to be intubated and ventilated. Apart from normally delivering a healthy baby 7 weeks ago she has no past medical history and is on no medication. She has never smoked and drinks approximately 8 units of alcohol per week, although she did not drink during her pregnancy. She is on no medication and there is no family history of heart disease.

Her echo shows poor left ventricular function with an ejection fraction of 25%. A still image is shown below:

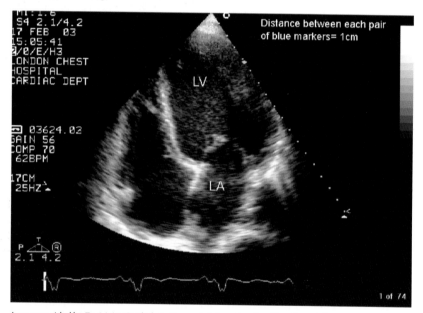

Image provided by Dr A Jain, Cardiology Research Fellow, London Chest Hospital, London

1   What is the most likely diagnosis?

- ☐ A Dilated cardiomyopathy due to alcohol
- ☐ B Post-viral dilated cardiomyopathy
- ☐ C Peripartum cardiomyopathy
- ☐ D Idiopathic dilated cardiomyopathy
- ☐ E Hypertrophic cardiomyopathy

Case 13

A 37-year-old patient with schizophrenia collapses on the psychiatric ward. Basic CPR is started by the nurses; when the arrest team arrive, the initial rhythm is found to be VF and he is cardioverted back to sinus rhythm and transferred to CCU. While he is on the ward he becomes unwell and arrests again, needing cardioversion (recorded rhythm strip shown below).

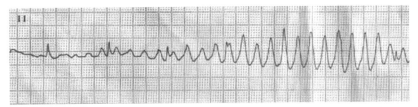

Image provided by Dr J Wilkinson, Cardiology Research Fellow, University College London, London

1   What does his ECG show?

- A   VF
- B   *Torsades de pointes*
- C   VT
- D   AF with bundle branch block
- E   Sinus rhythm with multiple ectopics

His resting ECG is shown below. His echocardiogram is normal and there was no troponin rise. Apart from smoking, he has no risk factors for ischaemic heart disease or significant past medical history. He was fit and active prior to this admission. All his electrolytes are normal. He is on numerous antipsychotic medications.

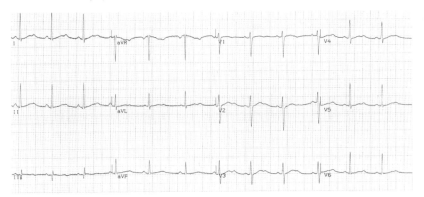

Image provided by Dr E Behr, Specialist Registrar in Cardiology, St George's Hospital, London

15

2 **Which of the following is most correct?**

☐ A He has congenital long QT syndrome
☐ B He has acquired long QT syndrome due to his neuroleptic medication
☐ C He has WPW syndrome
☐ D He has Brugada syndrome
☐ E He has right ventricular outflow tract (RVOT) dysplasia causing VT

Case 14

A 24-year-old man collapses without warning while rowing; by the time he gets to A&E he is in sinus rhythm and well. He is discharged from A&E with a diagnosis of vasovagal syncope. His GP notes that his cousin collapsed without prior symptoms at a similar age while playing football, and was dead on the side of the pitch by the time the ambulance arrived.

The GP orders an echocardiogram and the 2D image is shown below. You are told in the echo report that there are no abnormal gradients or valvular regurgitation on colour Doppler.

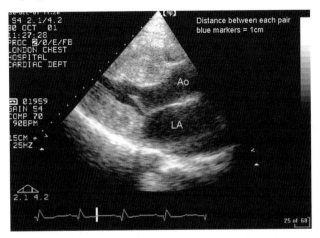

Image provided by Dr A Jain, Cardiology Research Fellow, London Chest Hospital, London

1   Which of the following statements is most accurate?

☐ A   His echocardiogram shows asymmetrical septal hypertrophy. The diagnosis is hypertrophic cardiomyopathy. He should be considered for an AICD insertion

☐ B   His echocardiogram shows asymmetrical septal hypertrophy. The diagnosis is hypertrophic cardiomyopathy. He should be put on a β-blocker and considered for a surgical myomectomy

☐ C   His echocardiogram shows asymmetrical septal hypertrophy. The diagnosis is hypertrophic cardiomyopathy. He should be put on amiodarone and followed up regularly in Outpatients

☐ D   His echocardiogram shows symmetrical septal hypertrophy. The diagnosis is hypertrophic cardiomyopathy. He should be put on a β-blocker and followed up regularly in outpatients

☐ E   His echocardiogram shows symmetrical septal hypertrophy consistent with athletic training and he should be reassured that he probably just had a faint due to hypoglycaemia

Case 15

You are referred an 84-year-old patient in A&E who is in pulmonary oedema that started suddenly at 4 am, waking her from her sleep. She has never had chest pain. She is normally fit and independent. However, she has recently been getting increasingly breathless walking to the shops and now needs to sleep with four pillows. She has been hypertensive for 20 years, but this has been controlled by her GP with a thiazide diuretic and, more recently, an ACE inhibitor as well. She is not diabetic and has never smoked.

Her BP is 120/80 mmHg, the JVP is raised and she has pitting oedema of her ankles. Her chest X-ray confirms your clinical findings of pulmonary oedema. Her ECG is shown below:

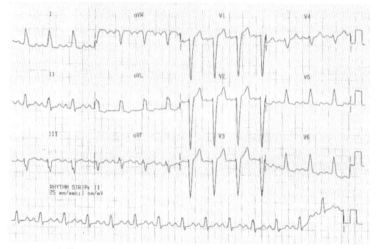

Image provided by Dr J Wilkinson, Cardiology Research Fellow, University College London, London

1   Which of the following statements is most accurate?

☐ A Her ECG shows left bundle branch block and she should receive thrombolysis immediately for an anterior MI

☐ B Her ECG shows slow VT and she should be started on amiodarone or cardioverted if she is haemodynamically compromised

☐ C Her ECG shows lateral ST depression and she should be treated as if she had acute coronary syndrome

☐ D Her ECG shows left bundle branch block and she should be treated for pulmonary oedema and considered for CPAP if she does not respond to the initial treatment

☐ E She has cardiogenic shock due to an anterior MI and should be referred for an urgent angiogram

Case 16

A 26-year-old man presents with a history of breathlessness and faints.

On examination the only finding is a long, soft, early diastolic murmur at the upper left sternal edge. He had corrective surgery for tetralogy of Fallot as a child. His ECG is shown below:

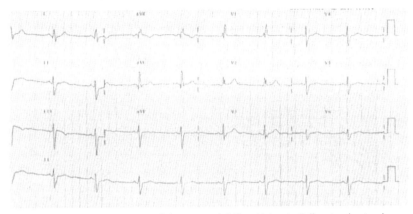

Image provided by Dr J Wilkinson, Cardiology Research Fellow, University College London, London

1   Which of the following statements is most accurate?

- [ ] A   His ECG is normal; he has a flow murmur from previous surgery. He is over-anxious as a result of his previous problems and should be reassured
- [ ] B   His ECG shows right bundle branch block; his murmur is likely to be due to pulmonary regurgitation but this is relatively benign and he can be reassured and does not need regular follow-up
- [ ] C   His ECG shows right bundle branch block and he probably has recurrent small pulmonary emboli causing his symptoms and ECG changes
- [ ] D   His ECG shows right bundle branch block; his murmur is likely to be due to pulmonary regurgitation. This can be associated with an increased risk of sudden death and he needs further investigation
- [ ] E   His ECG shows right bundle branch block; this is a normal variant and not related to his current presentation. His murmur is likely to be due to new aortic regurgitation, which is responsible for these symptoms and he should have an angiogram to assess this

Case 17

A 45-year-old builder is admitted with pulmonary oedema; he gives a history of worsening exercise tolerance over the past 6 months. He does not smoke and has no past medical history.

No evidence of ischaemic heart disease is found and he has an inpatient angiogram, which shows normal coronary arteries. He is apyrexial and all blood tests including CRP are normal. His subsequent chest X-ray is normal. Once his pulmonary oedema has resolved and he is well, he goes down for an echocardiogram, which is shown below (the lesion shown is demonstrated to be severe, by measurements not shown).

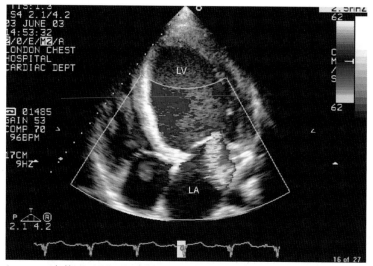

Image provided by Dr A Jain, Cardiology Research Fellow, London Chest Hospital, London

1   What is the best next step in his management?

- ☐   A   He has a ventricular septal defect and should have an intra-aortic balloon pump inserted and be referred for urgent surgery
- ☐   B   He has mitral regurgitation and should have a transoesophageal echocardiogram (TOE) to define the anatomy better. If possible, the first choice of treatment should be mitral valve repair
- ☐   C   He has mitral regurgitation and should have a TOE to define the anatomy better. If possible, the first choice of treatment should be mitral valve replacement with a non-mechanical valve, as he is a builder and wants to avoid warfarin and its potential complications
- ☐   D   He has mitral regurgitation and, although it is severe, his pulmonary oedema has resolved. He can be managed on medical therapy until his left ventricle is dilated
- ☐   E   He has aortic regurgitation and needs referral for a valve replacement

Case 18

A 56-year-old man with an MI is admitted to CCU on a Friday afternoon, after receiving thrombolysis, with tPA, in the A&E department. You are called to see him later (at 2 am) because he is breathless, has a low urine output and low BP (80/55 mmHg). He denies having chest pain but is sitting upright, very breathless, looking pale, sweaty and very unwell.

His ECG is shown below:

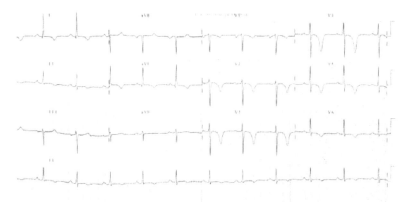

Image provided by Dr J Wilkinson, Cardiology Research Fellow, University College London, London

His chest X-ray is shown below:

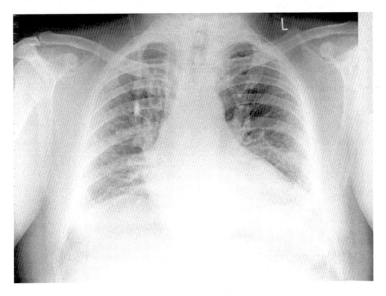

Image provided by Dr J Wilkinson, Cardiology Research Fellow, University College London, London

1   Which of the following statements is most appropriate?

☐   A   He has cardiogenic shock and should receive a second dose of thrombolysis before intubation and transfer to ICU for ventilation and further management

☐   B   He has cardiogenic shock; if possible, a Swan–Ganz catheter should be inserted to optimise his haemodynamics. He should have an urgent echo (if available) and you should consider insertion of an intra-aortic balloon pump, transferring him urgently to an intervention centre provided you can get him stable enough

☐   C   He has cardiogenic shock; if possible, a Swan–Ganz catheter should be inserted to optimise his haemodynamics. He should have an urgent echo (if available) and you should consider insertion of an intra-aortic balloon pump and transferring him to ICU, stabilising him for at least 48 hours before you consider transferring him to an intervention centre

☐   D   He has cardiogenic shock; he should have an urgent echo (if available) and you should start him on a high-dose, furosemide infusion, after an initial bolus of at least 200 mg, to treat his pulmonary oedema and help raise his urine output

☐   E   He has cardiogenic shock; if possible, a Swan–Ganz catheter should be inserted to optimise his haemodynamics. He should have an urgent echo (if available) and you should start him on inotropes and non-invasive ventilation, and get the cardiologists to review him urgently on Monday morning

Case 19

A 74-year-old lady is admitted with chest pain radiating to her left arm and generally feeling unwell.

Her chest is clear, oxygen saturations 100% on air and BP 130/84 mmHg. Her ECG is shown below:

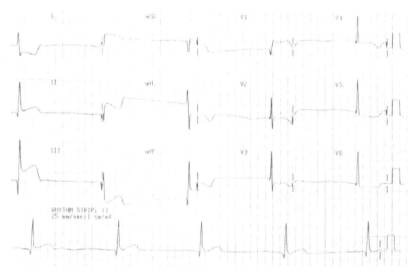

Image provided by Dr J Wilkinson, Cardiology Research Fellow, University College London, London

1   Which of the following statements is most appropriate?

☐   A   She has an inferior ST-elevation MI with complete heart block and needs to be taken to the angio suite for insertion of a temporary pacing wire

☐   B   She has an inferior ST-elevation MI with a sinus bradycardia and should be given thrombolysis and intravenous atropine

☐   C   She has an inferior ST-elevation MI with complete heart block and should be given thrombolysis as soon as possible

☐   D   She has an inferior ST-elevation MI with complete heart block and should be given thrombolysis as soon as possible and externally paced in the meantime

☐   E   She has complete heart block and should be referred for insertion of a permanent pacemaker

Case 20

The surgeons admit an 18-year-old man with suspected appendicitis. He is known to have long-standing congenital heart disease and has been on warfarin for many years. In view of this, the surgical nurses do an ECG on admission, which shows him to be in sinus rhythm. He is an intelligent young man and knows his condition well; he tells you he has had a procedure called a 'Fontan operation', where the vena cava is anastomosed directly to the pulmonary artery to bypass the pulmonary valve, and that he is regularly seen at a tertiary congenital heart disease unit. The surgical house officer has called you because the patient is complaining of palpitations.

His ECG is shown below. He is not haemodynamically compromised; BP 120/85 mmHg. His INR is 2.3.

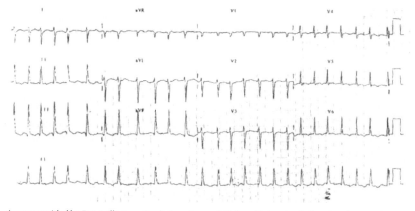

Image provided by Dr J Wilkinson, Cardiology Research Fellow, University College London, London

1 **Which of the following is the most appropriate next step?**

☐ A Arrange to cardiovert him; his arrhythmia is new-onset and he is already anticoagulated

☐ B Put him on digoxin to control his rate

☐ C Start him on an amiodarone infusion

☐ D Discuss his case with one of the cardiologists at his centre

☐ E Give him intravenous flecainide to terminate the rhythm

Case 21

The orthopaedic house officer asks you to see a 74-year-old patient who has become unwell with palpitations. He is known to have previously had an MI but has recently been fit and active. He is awaiting an elective knee replacement.

His ECG is shown below:

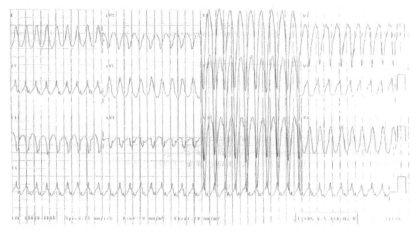

Image provided by Dr J Wilkinson, Cardiology Research Fellow, University College London, London

1   Which of the following is the correct diagnosis?

☐ A   Monomorphic ventricular tachycardia
☐ B   Polymorphic ventricular tachycardia
☐ C   Fast AF with underlying bundle branch block
☐ D   Sinus tachycardia with underlying bundle branch block
☐ E   *Torsades de pointes*

2   The patient looks unwell and has a blood pressure of 85/50 mmHg. How should he be managed?

☐ A   Put him on an amiodarone infusion
☐ B   You should arrange a semi-elective TOE and cardioversion
☐ C   Synchronised DC cardioversion
☐ D   He should be given intravenous digoxin and a heparin infusion
☐ E   He should be loaded with an oral β-blocker and put on a monitor

Case 22

The surgical house officer calls you. He is seeing a 68-year-old lady in his pre-clerking clinic; she is due to have a cholecystectomy. The patient has been complaining of palpitations for the last 2 days but this has not affected her exercise tolerance much. The house officer has done an ECG, which shows her to be in AF with a rate of 140 bpm. Her blood pressure is 133/75 mmHg. She is known to be mildly hypertensive, for which she is on bendroflumethiazide, but has no other medical problems and has never had an ECG before. The house officer is keen to cardiovert her and is already setting this up.

1   Which statement best describes how she should be managed?

- [ ] A   Because she is on a diuretic you need to check her potassium before she can have an anaesthetic for her cardioversion
- [ ] B   She should be anticoagulated with warfarin, have her rate controlled with medication, have an echocardiogram and be brought back for an elective cardioversion in 6–8 weeks
- [ ] C   She should be put on intravenous heparin and amiodarone and admitted to CCU
- [ ] D   She should be given aspirin and a β-blocker
- [ ] E   She should have carotid sinus massage and, failing this, intravenous adenosine

Case 23

You are asked to see a 34-year-old lady who has just arrived in the UK 6 weeks ago. She is 6 months pregnant and has become increasingly breathless on exertion over the last 5 months. She is now unable to walk up a single flight of stairs without having to stop three times.

The referring SHO can hear a soft murmur, which she thinks is diastolic. The left ventricular function is normal on echo.

Her ECG is shown below:

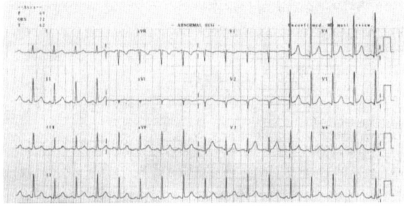

Image provided by Dr J Wilkinson, Cardiology Research Fellow, University College London, London

1   What is the most likely diagnosis?

- ☐ A   Peripartum cardiomyopathy
- ☐ B   Hypertrophic cardiomyopathy
- ☐ C   Recurrent pulmonary emboli
- ☐ D   Mitral stenosis
- ☐ E   Aortic regurgitation

Case 24

A 45-year-old lady presents with 3-week history of blackouts. She smokes but has no medical problems and is on no medication. She drinks 40 units of alcohol a week.

Her examination is normal.

Her echo is shown below:

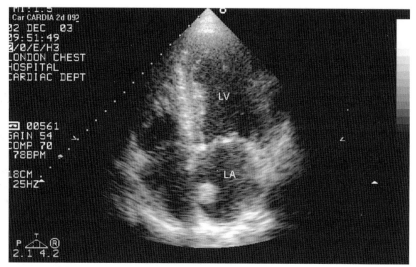

Image provided by Dr A Jain, Cardiology Research Fellow, London Chest Hospital, London

1   What is the diagnosis?

- ☐ A   Large atrial thrombus due to atrial fibrillation caused by excess alcohol
- ☐ B   Large atrial vegetation due to endocarditis
- ☐ C   Atrial myxoma
- ☐ D   Atrial fibroelastoma
- ☐ E   Atrial haematoma

Case 25

The surgical house officer asks you how to manage a patient's anticoagulation. He is due to have an elective hernia repair and is on warfarin for a ball-and-cage (Starr–Edwards) mechanical mitral valve.

INR   3.5

1   What do you advise?

☐ A   Stop the warfarin 5 days before the operation and start aspirin cover

☐ B   Stop the warfarin 3 days before the operation and restart it a day after the operation

☐ C   Stop the warfarin 5 days before the operation and ask the GP to provide low molecular weight heparin cover (daily injections)

☐ D   Omit warfarin the day before the operation, then on the day of the operation check the clotting early and give 1mg of vitamin K and FFP (as necessary), checking the INR every 30 minutes till $\leqslant 1.2$. Restart the warfarin 72 hours after the operation and titrate to the desired INR

☐ E   Stop warfarin 4 days before the operation; admit the patient the next day and put them on a full therapeutic dose of intravenous heparin. Stop the heparin 4 hours prior to the surgery, then restart it afterwards; keep the patient on heparin until they are back on warfarin and the desired INR is reached

Case 26

The nurse on CCU calls you to discuss a 45-year-old man who was admitted 6 hours ago and received thrombolysis for an anterior MI. The nurse is concerned that the patient is having frequent ectopics and episodes of bigeminy on the monitor. You reassure her that his electrolytes are all normal and that no further action is necessary; she is not happy and insists you come and see the patient and start an anti-arrhythmic.

On examination the patient is asymptomatic with a normal examination; the only abnormality you see is that his blood sugar is 12 mmol/L (he is not known to be diabetic). His monitor shows ventricular ectopics and episodes of bigeminy.

1   What is the most appropriate course of action?

- ☐ A   Reassure the nurse that no further action is necessary
- ☐ B   Start an intravenous magnesium and potassium infusion
- ☐ C   Reassure the nurse that no anti-arrhythmics are necessary, but that an insulin sliding scale should be started
- ☐ D   Put the patient on intravenous amiodarone and an insulin sliding scale
- ☐ E   Start the patient on oral potassium supplements and metformin

Case 27

A 44-year-old man presents with 3-week history of increasing breathlessness. He gives a background of feeling generally unwell, with weight loss, night sweats and malaise over the last 4 months. He has never smoked, has no other medical problems and is on no medication.

On examination he is sitting up, unwell and very breathless at rest, BP 100/50 mmHg, pulse 110 bpm, sinus rhythm. He has splinter haemorrhages on four of his fingernails and is pyrexial. On auscultation, he has crepitations in his mid-zones and his oxygen saturations are 88% on 2L oxygen. He has a collapsing pulse and a long diastolic murmur. His ECG is normal.

1   What is the most appropriate management?

- [ ] A   Arrange for an intra-aortic balloon pump to be inserted to support his circulation and arrange a cardiothoracic surgical review
- [ ] B   Start non-invasive ventilation and arrange an urgent echocardiogram and cardiology review
- [ ] C   Arrange for an intra-aortic balloon pump to be inserted to support his circulation, start non-invasive ventilation and arrange a cardiothoracic surgical review
- [ ] D   Call anaesthetists to intubate the patient and fast-bleep the cardiothoracic surgeons
- [ ] E   Give the patient intravenous furosemide and an ACE inhibitor for his cardiac failure

Case 28

An 80-year-old lady presents with a 2-week history of malaise, fever and vomiting. She has no other symptoms.

Her temperature is 37.5 °C and apart from her being emaciated and frail with a soft apical pansystolic murmur, no other abnormalities are found on examination. Her chest X-ray is normal. She has never seen a doctor before now and is on no medication. Her full blood count shows her to have a microcytic anaemia; her biochemistry is normal.

1   What is the most appropriate management?

☐ A   Start her on intravenous antibiotics for endocarditis, book a TOE and admit her

☐ B   Start her on intravenous antibiotics for endocarditis, book a transthoracic echo and admit her

☐ C   Stix test her urine and send off an MSU; consider antibiotics, depending on the result, and admit her for further investigation

☐ D   Send off at least three sets of blood cultures, start her on intravenous antibiotics for endocarditis, book a transthoracic echo and admit her

☐ E   Send off at least three sets of blood cultures, start her on intravenous antibiotics for endocarditis, book a TOE and admit her

Case 29

Four weeks after having had a prosthetic aortic valve inserted (for calcific aortic stenosis), a 60-year-old man presents with a 2-week history of malaise and fevers. He is on warfarin but no other medication and has no other medical history. He has no other symptoms.

His temperature is 38.5 °C; apart from two splinters on his right first finger (he is a carpenter), no other abnormalities are found on examination and you can hear no murmurs. His chest X-ray is normal. His stix urinalysis is normal.

1   What is the most appropriate management?

- [ ] A   Start him on intravenous antibiotics for endocarditis and arrange a cardiology opinion as soon as possible
- [ ] B   Take blood cultures and admit him for observation but do not start antibiotics until you know what organism you are dealing with
- [ ] C   Take blood cultures and send him home with a week's supply of oral antibiotics, recheck his bloods in 1 week
- [ ] D   Take blood cultures, start him on intravenous antibiotics for endocarditis, ensure his anticoagulation is therapeutic and arrange a cardiology opinion as soon as possible
- [ ] E   Reassure him that a minor fever after major surgery is common and send him home

Case 30

A medical house officer asks you to explain the following cardiac catheter results of a young child who becomes breathless and cyanosed on exertion:

	O$_2$ Saturation, %	Pressure, mmHg
Right atrium	60	6
Right ventricle	75	85
Pulmonary artery	75	20
PA wedge		12
Left ventricle	100	90
Aorta	100	90

1   What is the diagnosis?

☐ A   VSD
☐ B   VSD with Eisenmenger's
☐ C   Tetralogy of Fallot
☐ D   Pulmonary atresia
☐ E   Pulmonary regurgitation

Case 31

You are asked to review a 40-year-old man. He was admitted with a 12-week history of fevers, malaise and weight loss. He had a Starr–Edwards aortic valve replacement 15 years ago, for which he is on warfarin, but has no other medical history. He was admitted 4 days ago with a fever and transient ischaemic attack (TIA), from which he has made a full recovery. The admitting team started him on intravenous antibiotics for endocarditis. His echocardiogram clearly shows a structure that is consistent with a small vegetation on his aortic valve; the valve is functioning normally and there are no other abnormalities. His last check-up echo, a year ago, was normal. His initial four sets of blood cultures have come back showing no growth at 48 hours; the admitting team are now questioning their diagnosis.

The patient is feeling better and apart from a few splinter haemorrhages you find no abnormalities on examination. His CT head is normal.

1   What is the most appropriate course of action?

- [ ] A   Stop the antibiotics and reculture if he spikes another fever
- [ ] B   Start antifungal cover
- [ ] C   Speak to the microbiologists and say you suspect an atypical organism (HACEK), and ask them to look for this and check whether your current therapy covers these organisms
- [ ] D   Arrange a TOE to confirm or refute the diagnosis
- [ ] E   Arrange a lupus screen to rule out Libman–Sacks endocarditis

Case 32

You are asked to see a 33-year-old man. He has had increasing problems with his walking since he was 11. He has dysarthria and nystagmus. He has become increasingly breathless over the last 6 weeks.

On examination he clearly has cardiac failure but no murmurs. His chest X-ray shows cardiomegaly and pulmonary oedema.

1   What is the most likely diagnosis?

☐   A   Post-viral cardiomyopathy
☐   B   Acute pericarditis
☐   C   Constrictive pericarditis
☐   D   Duchenne muscular dystrophy
☐   E   Friedreich's ataxia

Case 33

You are asked to review a 28-year-old afro-carribean lady. She was admitted a week ago with aortic valve endocarditis (confirmed on blood cultures and TOE) and had been improving on intravenous antibiotics. She is known to have a bicuspid aortic valve. She is feeling increasingly generally unwell and has started spiking fevers. Her current ECG is shown below, it was reported as normal on admission. Her white count and CRP have risen.

Her ECG is shown below (admission ECG was normal):

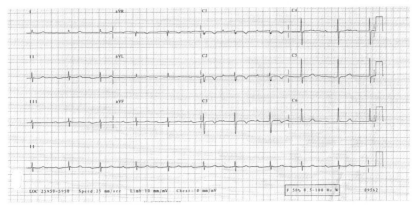

Image provided by Dr A Jain, Cardiology Research Fellow, London Chest Hospital, London

1   What is the most likely diagnosis?

- A   Reassure the nursing staff that this is a normal variant
- B   Take further blood cultures and reassure the nursing staff that this is a normal variant
- C   Change her antibiotics
- D   Take further blood cultures and organise another TOE
- E   Take further blood cultures and organise a CT scan

Case 34

A 46-year-old lady is admitted with a myocardial infarction.

You notice a cutaneous abnormality (which is shown below); no other abnormalities are found on examination.

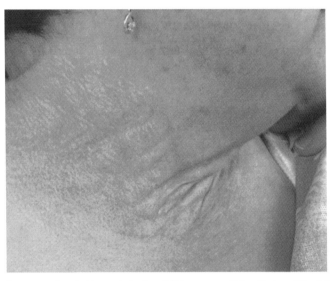

Image reproduced with permission from Self-Asssessment Colour Review of Cardiology, *Stuart D. Rosen et al., 1997, Manson Publishing: London*

1   What is the diagnosis?

- ☐ A   Pseudoxanthoma elasticum
- ☐ B   Ehlers–Danlos syndrome
- ☐ C   Xanthomata
- ☐ D   Marfan's syndrome
- ☐ E   Tangier disease

Case 35

A 26-year-old man presents with an 8-week history of increasing breathlessness on exertion. He has no past medical history and is not on any drugs.

His left ventricular function is normal on echocardiogram. His cardiac catheter data are shown below:

	Saturation, %	Systolic/Diastolic Pressure, mmHg
Right atrium	50	20/13
Right ventricle	50	122/15
Pulmonary artery	50	128/81
PA wedge		Not obtainable
Left ventricle	95	130/2 (LVEDP 5)
Aorta	95	100/70

1   Which of the following is not a treatment option?

- A   Intravenous epoprostenol (prostacyclin)
- B   Cardiac transplantation
- C   Sildenafil
- D   Percutaneous device closure
- E   Diltiazem

Case 36

A 26-year-old lady is referred to a cardiologist after her GP heard a murmur when she was 'booking in', 8 weeks pregnant. She has no past medical history and is on no medication.

Her cardiac catheter data are shown below:

	O$_2$ Saturation, %	Pressure, mmHg
IVC	65	
Right atrium	80	5
Right ventricle	80	30
Pulmonary artery	80	30
PA wedge		12
Left ventricle	100	100
Aorta	100	95

1   What is the most likely diagnosis?

☐ A   Aortic stenosis
☐ B   Atrial septal defect (ASD)
☐ C   Normal haemodynamics for pregnancy
☐ D   Patent ductus arteriosus (PDA)
☐ E   VSD

Case 37

A 66-year-old lady presents to your clinic with increasing breathlessness on exertion over a 3-month period. Her only past medical history is that she has been followed up by the haematologists for Waldenström's macroglobulinaemia for the last few years.

On examination her BP is 125/84 mmHg, she has an irregular heart rhythm, her JVP is raised to her ears and she has some pitting ankle oedema. Her chest is clear. Her chest X-ray shows a normal-sized heart and clear lung fields. Her ECG shows her to be in AF with a rate of 130 bpm. Her echocardiogram shows normal LV and RV systolic function but thickened myocardium with a speckled pattern.

1   Which of the following is the best treatment option?

- ☐ A   Load her with oral digoxin to control her heart rate
- ☐ B   Start her on flecainide
- ☐ C   Cardiovert her immediately
- ☐ D   Start her on a β-blocker to control her heart rate
- ☐ E   Try carotid sinus massage

Case 38

A 57-year-old man presents with severe, tearing, central chest pain radiating to his back. He is a lifelong asthmatic and smoker. He was diagnosed as hypertensive 2 years ago but has no other medical problems. He is on a salbutamol inhaler (as required), aspirin and bendroflumethiazide.

On examination he is pale and in pain. BP right arm 100/45 mmHg, left arm 155/95 mmHg; he has a soft early diastolic murmur; his chest is clear; and no other abnormalities are found. His ECG shows 2-mm ST elevation in leads II, III and aVF.

1   Which of the following is the best treatment option?

- [ ] A   He should be given thrombolysis
- [ ] B   He should be referred for primary angioplasty
- [ ] C   He should be put an a labetalol infusion and have either a TOE or a CT chest with contrast
- [ ] D   He should be given a nitrate infusion and thrombolysis
- [ ] E   He should be put an a nitrate infusion and have either a TOE or a CT chest with contrast

Case 39

You review a 73-year-old man in Outpatients. He had a large anterior MI a year ago for which he was treated with thrombolysis. He gets out of breath walking up an incline but has not had chest pain since his original MI. He is on atenolol, aspirin and simvastatin.

Coronary angiography (done 2 weeks ago) shows a blocked mid left anterior descending artery with retrograde filling of the distal vessels and good collaterals. His dominant right coronary artery and the left circumflex artery are unobstructed. There is akinesia of the anterior wall and only moderate left ventricular function; his LV is not dilated.

1   Which of the following best describes the regime he should be on?

- ☐ A   Add spironolactone to his current medication
- ☐ B   Switch his atenolol to bisoprolol, start him on ramipril and spironolactone
- ☐ C   Add spironolactone and ramipril to his current medication
- ☐ D   Add spironolactone, clopidogrel and ramipril to his current medication
- ☐ E   Switch his atenolol to bisoprolol and start him on ramipril

Case 40

You are fast-bleeped to the resuscitation room in A&E by the SHO. A 76-year-old man has palpitations; he has no other symptoms and does not feel particularly unwell. He is known to have ischaemic heart disease. His blood pressure is normal and he is sitting up chatting. On seeing his ECG, the nurses rushed him round to the resuscitation room and persuaded the SHO to fast-bleep you. The patient looks slightly perplexed but not unwell.

His ECG is shown below:

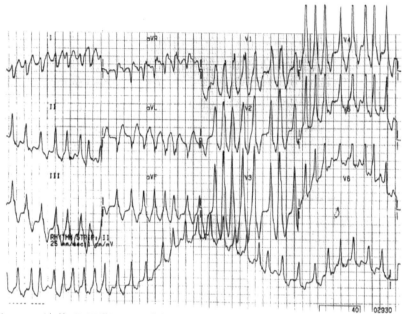

Image provided by Dr J Wilkinson, Cardiology Research Fellow, University College London, London

1   What is the next step?

- ☐ A   Fast-bleep the anaesthetist and cardiovert the patient as soon as they arrive
- ☐ B   Insert a central line and start intravenous amiodarone
- ☐ C   Give a trial of intravenous adenosine
- ☐ D   Start him on oral digoxin
- ☐ E   Start him on an intravenous magnesium infusion

Chapter Two

RESPIRATORY MEDICINE

Case 1

A 41-year-old man was referred to the hospital with a 1-week history of fever, malaise, increasing confusion, cough and breathlessness. The cough was initially dry but has become productive of yellow sputum in the last few days. He saw the GP 4 days ago, who prescribed amoxicillin with no benefit. His wife reports that he has also been suffering from abdominal pain and vomiting. He is a smoker of 20/day and works in a large law firm.

On examination, he looks unwell and dehydrated. Temperature 39 °C, BP 100/50 mmHg, pulse 120 bpm, respiratory rate 30/min, SpO$_2$ 89% on air and Glasgow Coma Scale (GCS) score 12. Auscultation of his chest reveals crackles in the left lower zone. His abdomen is generally tender on palpation. Examination is otherwise unremarkable.

Urinalysis   Blood ++

Investigations:

Hb	11.1 g/dL
WCC	10.6 × 10^9/L
Neutrophils	9.2 × 10^9/L
Platelets	151 × 10^9/L
Sodium	127 mmol/L
Potassium	3.4 mmol/L
Urea	9.0 mmol/L
Creatinine	120 μmol/L
Bilirubin	28 μmol/L
AST	220 U/L
ALT	190 U/L
ALP	140 U/L
Albumin	28 g/L
CRP	110 mg/L

Arterial blood gases (ABG) on air:
pH	7.39
PCO$_2$	4.66 kPa
PO$_2$	7.3 kPa
Bicarbonate	21.4 mmol/L

1   Which organism is most likely to be responsible?

☐   A   *Streptococcus pneumoniae*
☐   B   *Legionella pneumophila*
☐   C   *Mycoplasma pneumoniae*
☐   D   *Coxiella burnetii*
☐   E   *Chlamydia psittaci*

2   Which investigation would confirm the diagnosis quickly?

☐   A   Blood culture
☐   B   Urinary *Legionella* antigen
☐   C   Acute and convalescent atypical serology
☐   D   Sputum for Gram stain
☐   E   Cold agglutinins

Case 2

A 19-year-old man presented with a 10-day history of headaches and malaise. He then developed a dry cough and breathlessness and was admitted to hospital.

On examination he was pyrexial, and had a rash (see below).

Investigations:

Hb	9.4 g/dL
WCC	10×10^9/L
Neutrophils	9.2×10^9/L
Platelets	200×10^9/L
Reticulocytes	5.1%
Sodium	129 mmol/L
Potassium	5.0 mmol/L
Urea	4.4 mmol/L
Creatinine	90 µmol/L
Bilirubin	30 µmol/L
AST	44 U/L
ALT	30 U/L
ALP	121 U/L
Albumin	35 g/L
LDH	495 U/L

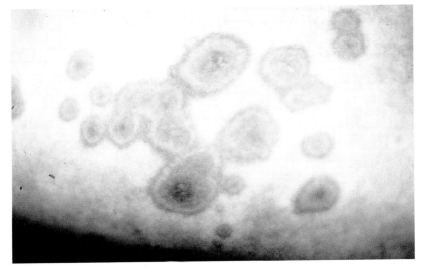

Image courtesy of Dr M Ardern-Jones, John Radcliffe Hospital, Oxford

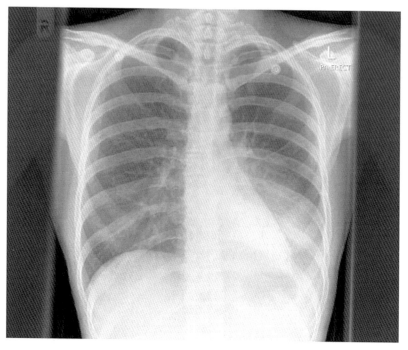

1   What is the diagnosis?

- [ ] A   Epstein–Barr virus (EBV)
- [ ] B   *Legionella* pneumonia
- [ ] C   Streptococcal pneumonia
- [ ] D   Tuberculosis
- [ ] E   *Mycoplasma* pneumonia

2   What two tests would help you confirm the diagnosis?

- [ ] A   Blood cultures
- [ ] B   Arterial blood gases
- [ ] C   *Mycoplasma* serology
- [ ] D   Cold agglutinins
- [ ] E   Indirect Coombs' test
- [ ] F   *Legionella* antigen
- [ ] G   EBV serology
- [ ] H   Sputum culture
- [ ] I   High-resolution CT scan

Case 3

A 54-year-old stonemason was referred to the clinic with a 3-year history of progressive breathlessness. He is an ex-smoker (40 pack-years) having stopped 14 years ago.

On examination he looked well, was not clubbed and there was no lymphadenopathy. His chest was hyperexpanded and he had basal inspiratory crackles.

His spirometry revealed:

FEV_1	38% predicted
FVC	70% predicted
K_{CO}	55% predicted

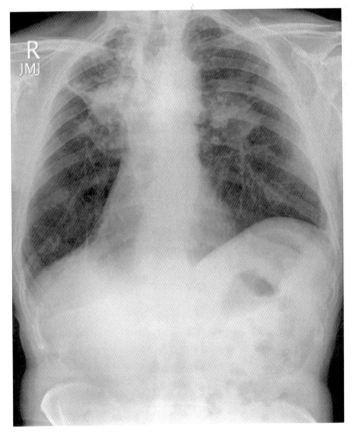

1   What is the underlying diagnosis?

- [ ] A Silicosis
- [ ] B Asbestosis
- [ ] C Byssinosis
- [ ] D Berylliosis
- [ ] E Simple pneumoconiosis

Three years later he presented to A&E with increasing shortness of breath, cough and wheeze. Over the last year he had recurrent chest infections and now had a cough productive of green sputum.

On examination: respiratory rate 30/min, temperature 36.2 °C, BP 160/100 mmHg, pulse 130 bpm, SpO_2 57% on air. He was breathing through pursed lips. Auscultation of his chest revealed expiratory wheeze and crackles throughout.

Blood gases on 28% oxygen:

pH	7.22
PO_2	7.9 kPa
PCO_2	8.0 kPa
Bicarbonate	20 mmol/L
Base excess	−3

2   What do the blood gases show?

- [ ] A Metabolic acidosis
- [ ] B Respiratory acidosis
- [ ] C Mixed respiratory and metabolic acidosis
- [ ] D Respiratory acidosis with metabolic compensation
- [ ] E Metabolic acidosis with respiratory compensation

Despite controlled oxygen, antibiotics, nebulisers and hydrocortisone, he fails to improve and is moved to ICU where he is started on non-invasive ventilation (inspiratory positive airway pressure, IPAP, 12 cmH_2O; and expiratory positive airway pressure, EPAP, 5 cmH_2O).

Initially he does very well but he suddenly desaturates, although his BP remains stable.

On examianation the left side of his chest had reduced expansion, was hyper-resonant on percussion with diminished breath sounds. The trachea was not deviated.

3   **What would you do?**

☐   A   Aspirate left side of the chest with a 16- or 14-G cannula – maximum 2 litres
☐   B   Insert a left-sided chest drain
☐   C   Remove non-invasive ventilation
☐   D   Increase IPAP
☐   E   Reduce EPAP

Case 4

A 70-year-old lady presented in acute respiratory distress. She had had some chest pain earlier that morning. She is an ex-smoker of 30 pack-years (20/day for 30 years).

On examination she looked unwell. Respiratory rate 30/min, pulse 120 bpm, BP 80/50 mmHg and O_2 saturation was 80% on air. Heart sounds were normal and her chest was clear.

ABG on air:

pH	7.44
PO_2	7.0 kPa
PCO_2	3.25 kPa
Base excess	−2.6
Bicarbonate	19.5 mmol/L

You manage to get an urgent CT within the hour, shown below:

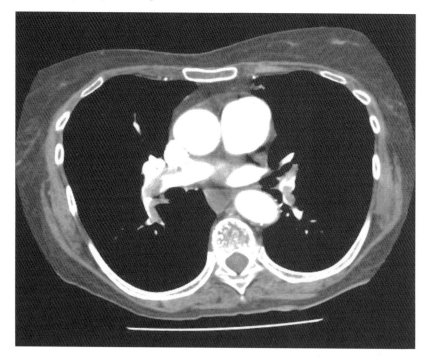

1   What is the diagnosis?

☐   A   Congestive cardiac failure
☐   B   Myocardial infarction
☐   C   Pneumonia
☐   D   Pulmonary embolism (PE)
☐   E   Pneumothorax

2   The patient deteriorates; what is the immediate management?

☐   A   Diuretics
☐   B   Intravenous antibiotics
☐   C   Streptokinase
☐   D   Alteplase
☐   E   Low molecular weight heparin

Case 5

You are on call on Boxing Day and you are referred a 61-year-old lady with shortness of breath. Her only other complaint is of recent diarrhoea. She is a smoker of 30/day.

On examination she looks unwell. Her temperature is 38.5 °C. On auscultation of her chest she has coarse crackles at the right base. She has a distended abdomen with dullness in the flanks.

Investigations show:

Hb	11.1 g/dL
WCC	12.3×10^9/L
Neutrophils	9.5×10^9/L
Platelets	88×10^9/L
MCV	101 fL
Sodium	130 mmol/L
Potassium	3.4 mmol/L
Urea	7.8 mmol/L
Creatinine	77 μmol/L
INR	1.4
Bilirubin	16 μmol/L
AST	73 U/L
ALP	300 U/L
Albumin	30 g/L
γGT	100 U/L
Creatine kinase	700 U/L

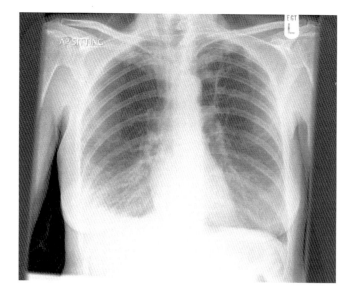

1   The most likely diagnosis is?

- [ ] A *Mycoplasma* pneumonia
- [ ] B *Legionella* pneumonia
- [ ] C Aspiration pneumonia
- [ ] D Streptococcal pneumonia
- [ ] E *Klebsiella* pneumonia

Case 6

A 39-year-old Irish accountant was referred to the clinic with a 4-month history of progressive breathlessness. He noticed this mainly on climbing the stairs. Over the last few months he had been using some eye drops from the local pharmacy for dry eyes. He was also complaining of fatigue, night sweats and polyuria. He was a non-smoker and drank 20 units of alcohol a week.

On examination he had conjunctival injection, but examination of his eyes was otherwise unremarkable. He had no rash or joint swelling. On auscultation of his chest he had fine inspiratory crackles. Heart sounds were normal. He had no organomegaly on palpation of the abdomen. Urinalysis was unremarkable.

Investigations:

Hb	10.1 g/dL
MCV	84 fL
WCC	6.4×10^9/L
Platelets	201×10^9/L
ESR	45 mm/h
Sodium	141 mmol/L
Potassium	3.9 mmol/L
Urea	7.2 mmol/L
Creatinine	100 μmol/L
Bilirubin	23 μmol/L
AST	51 U/L
ALP	191 U/L
Albumin	45 g/L
Tuberculin test	Negative

Pulmonary function tests:
FEV_1	75% predicted
FVC	70% predicted
T_{LCO}	80% predicted

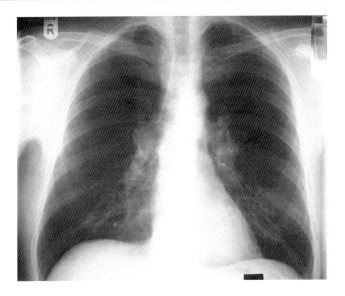

1   What is the most likely diagnosis?

☐ A Tuberculosis
☐ B Berylliosis
☐ C Small-cell lung carcinoma
☐ D Sarcoidosis
☐ E Langerhans' cell histiocytosis

2   Which of the following is most likely to give you a definitive diagnosis?

☐ A Serum angiotensin-coverting enzyme (ACE)
☐ B Sputum for microbiology
☐ C Bronchoscopy and transbronchial biopsies
☐ D Bronchoscopy and endobronchial biopsies
☐ E Kveim test

Case 7

A 16-year-old boy presents to Outpatients having coughed up a small amount of bright-red blood. He is mildly short of breath and feels 'wheezy'. His mother says he has always been a 'chesty' child. He was teased at school as he has always been the smallest in his class. His brother and sister were fit and well. He had a dog at home.

On examination he looked well and was not breathless at rest. He had clubbing. He had nasal polyps and auscultation of his chest revealed coarse crackles throughout both lung fields. His abdomen was distended but soft.

Urinalysis	Protein	+
	Glucose	++
	Nitrites	Negative
	Leucocytes	Negative

Investigations:

Hb	11.0 g/dL
WCC	12.1 × 10^9/L ↑
Neutrophils	91%
Lymphocytes	8%
Monocytes	0.4%
MCV	84 fL
Platelets	450 × 10^9/L ↑
ESR	35 mm/h ↑
CRP	40 mg/L ↑
Sodium	137 mmol/L
Potassium	3.9 mmol/L
Urea	6.4 mmol/L
Creatinine	62 μmol/L ↓
Bilirubin	31 μmol/L ↑
AST	46 U/L ↑
ALP	221 U/L ↑
Albumin	38 g/L
Protein	74 g/L
Magnesium	0.64 mmol/L
Calcium	2.1 mmol/L
Phosphate	0.75 mmol/L

Spirometry:

FEV$_1$	60% predicted
FVC	80% predicted
PEF	350 L/min
KCO	70% predicted

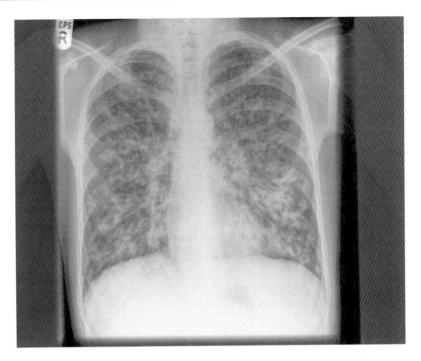

1   What is the most likely underlying diagnosis?

☐   A   Cystic fibrosis
☐   B   Kartagener's syndrome
☐   C   Asthma
☐   D   Allergic bronchopulmonary aspergillosis
☐   E   Goodpasture's syndrome

2   What test is most likely to establish a diagnosis?

☐   A   Methacholine challenge test
☐   B   Anti-GBM antibodies
☐   C   Electron microscopy of cilia
☐   D   Sweat test
☐   E   *Aspergillus* precipitins

3   Which pathogen is most likely to colonise this patient?

☐   A   *Streptococcus pneumoniae*
☐   B   *Staphylococcus aureus*
☐   C   *Aspergillus fumigatus*
☐   D   *Pseudomonas aeruginosa*
☐   E   *Mycobacterium tuberculosis*

Case 8

A 56-year-old man presented to his GP with a 4-week history of feeling generally unwell. He described nasal congestion, with pain under his left eye, flu-like symptoms and lethargy. His GP made a diagnosis of sinusitis and gave him a course of antibiotics. He did not improve and developed breathlessness, cough and chest pain. He had previously been fit and his only past medical history was of an inguinal hernia repair 10 years previously. He worked in a shop. He smoked 10 cigarettes a day and drank about 10 units of alcohol a week. He was taking no regular medication.

On examination he looked unwell and pale. Observations: respiratory rate 34/min, BP 140/85 mmHg, pulse 120 bpm, temperature 36.6 °C. He had crusting of his nasal septum. His JVP was not elevated; heart sounds were normal. Auscultation of his chest revealed fine crackles bilaterally. His abdominal and neurological examinations were unremarkable.

Urinalysis	Protein	++
	Blood	++
	Nitrites	Negative
	Leucocytes	Negative
	Bilirubin	Negative

Investigations:

Hb	8.1 g/dL ↓
WBC	6.3 × 10⁹/L
MCV	81 fL
Platelets	510 × 10⁹/L ↑
ESR	114 mm/h ↑
CRP	45 mg/L ↑
Sodium	142 mmol/L
Potassium	5.9 mmol/L ↑
Urea	21 mmol/L ↑
Creatinine	341 µmol/L ↑
Bilirubin	18 µmol/L ↑
AST	31 U/L
ALP	191 U/L ↑
Albumin	34 g/L ↓

Spirometry:

FEV$_1$	72% predicted
FVC	77% predicted
K$_{CO}$	122% predicted

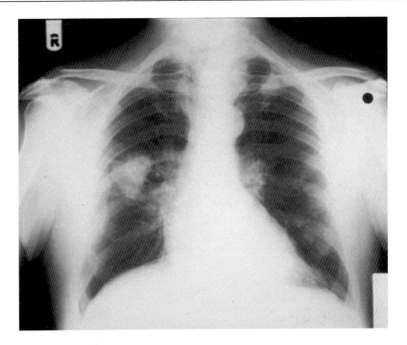

1   What is the least likely diagnosis?

- [ ] A   Wegener's granulomatosis
- [ ] B   Microscopic polyangiitis
- [ ] C   Goodpasture's syndrome/anti-GBM disease
- [ ] D   Pulmonary oedema
- [ ] E   *Legionella* pneumonia

2   What is the most likely diagnosis?

- [ ] A   Wegener's granulomatosis
- [ ] B   Microscopic polyangiitis
- [ ] C   Goodpasture's syndrome/anti-GBM disease
- [ ] D   Pulmonary oedema
- [ ] E   *Legionella* pneumonia

3   Which investigation would help make a diagnosis?

- [ ] A   c-ANCA (anti-proteinase 3)
- [ ] B   Anti-GBM antibodies
- [ ] C   p-ANCA (anti-myeloperoxidase)
- [ ] D   *Legionella* antigen
- [ ] E   Echocardiogram

4   How would you treat this patient?

☐   A   Intravenous antibiotics
☐   B   Intravenous diuretics
☐   C   Cyclophosphamide and prednisolone
☐   D   Methylprednisolone and methotrexate
☐   E   Plasmapheresis

Case 9

A 39-year-old man presented to his general practitioner with a 3-month history of fever, rhinitis and weight loss. Two weeks ago he had an exacerbation of asthma and was treated with a course erythromycin. He also complained of weakness in his hands and legs. He has a past medical history of angina. He is an ex-smoker and stopped 5 years ago.

On examination he has a rash over his shins – see below. Auscultation of his chest reveals a mild expiratory wheeze. Examination was otherwise unremarkable. Urinalysis was normal.

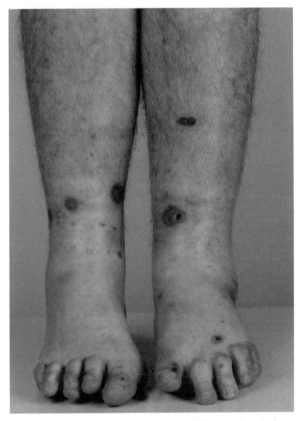

Image courtesy of Dr M Ardern-Jones, John Radcliffe Hospital, Oxford

Investigations:

Hb	12.1 g/dL
MCV	84 fL
WCC	9.4×10^9/L
Neutrophils	5.3×10^9/L
Lymphocytes	1.8×10^9/L
Monocytes	0.3×10^9/L
Basophils	0.08×10^9/L
Platelets	411×10^9/L
ESR	82 mm/h
Sodium	138 mmol/L
Potassium	4.2 mmol/L
Urea	4.1 mmol/L
Creatinine	111 µmol/L

1   What is the diagnosis?

☐ A Microscopic polyangiitis
☐ B Wegener's granulomatosis
☐ C Eosinophilic pneumonia secondary to erythromycin
☐ D Churg–Strauss syndrome
☐ E Allergic bronchopulmonary aspergillosis

2   Which two of the following investigations would aid diagnosis?

☐ A c-ANCA
☐ B p-ANCA-positive, anti-myeloperoxidase (MPO) antibody-positive
☐ C p-ANCA-positive, anti-myeloperoxidase-negative
☐ D Positive skin test/radioallergosorbent test (RAST) for *Aspergillus fumigatus*
☐ E Renal biopsy
☐ F Bronchoscopy alone
☐ G Bronchoscopy and bronchoalveolar lavage
☐ H Methacholine challenge test

Case 10

A 55-year-old asthmatic patient presented in December with increasing cough and wheeze. She described a cough productive of brown sputum. She had no other past medical history. She was taking a steroid inhaler regularly and increasing doses of β-agonist with no alleviation of her symptoms. She worked in a bakery for many years. She is an ex-smoker and stopped smoking 20 years ago. She has a dog at home.

On examination she had a temperature of 38 °C. She was breathless at rest. She had reduced expansion anteriorly on the left side, with corresponding reduced breath sounds. She had a mild expiratory wheeze.

Investigations:

Hb	14.1 g/dL
WCC	12.7 × 10⁹/L ↑
Neutrophils,	7.37 × 10⁹/L
Lymphocytes	2.55 × 10⁹/L
Monocytes	0.6 × 10⁹/L
Basophils	0.05 × 10⁹/L
MCV	87.3 fL
Platelets	314 × 10⁹/L
ESR	28 mm/h ↑
CRP	16 mg/L ↑
Sodium	138 mmol/L
Potassium	4.9 mmol/L
Urea	4.8 mmol/L
Creatinine	95 µmol/L
Bilirubin	12 µmol/L
ALT	49 U/L ↑
ALP	61 U/L
Albumin	36 g/L

Chest X-rays, 1 month apart, the first on presentation, are shown overleaf:

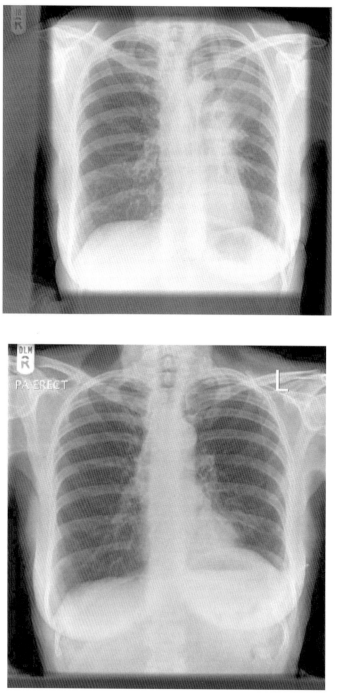

1   What does the first chest X-ray show?

- [ ] A   Left upper lobe consolidation
- [ ] B   Left upper lobe collapse
- [ ] C   Left lower lobe collapse
- [ ] D   Left lower lobe consolidation
- [ ] E   Lingular consolidation

2   What is the diagnosis?

- [ ] A   Occupational asthma
- [ ] B   Exacerbation of asthma
- [ ] C   Allergic bronchopulmonary aspergillosis
- [ ] D   Churg–Strauss syndrome
- [ ] E   Loeffler's syndrome

3   What investigation would help make a diagnosis?

- [ ] A   p-ANCA
- [ ] B   c-ANCA
- [ ] C   Positive skin test/radioallergosorbent test for *Aspergillus fumigatus*
- [ ] D   Methacholine challenge test
- [ ] E   Lung function tests

Case 11

A 67-year-old non-smoker was referred to the respiratory consultant with a 3-month history of progressive shortness of breath. She was also complaining of right-sided chest pain, which she described as a constant severe ache. She had lost about 5 kg in the last month and felt lethargic. She had initially put the symptoms down to the stress of recently being widowed. Her husband, who used to work as a plumber, died of a 'lung problem'. She has never worked outside the home, and has two daughters who are fit and well.

On examination she looked unwell and was breathless at rest. Examination of her chest revealed reduced expansion, percussion note, vocal fremitus and breath sounds throughout the right hemithorax.

Investigations:

Hb	10.2 g/dL
WCC	10.8×10^9/L
MCV	81 fL
Platelets	471×10^9/L
ESR	69 mm/h
CRP	44 mg/L
Sodium	136 mmol/L
Potassium	3.7 mmol/L
Urea	6.6 mmol/L
Creatinine	77 µmol/L
Bilirubin	34 µmol/L
AST	21 U/L
ALP	97 U/L
Albumin	37 g/L

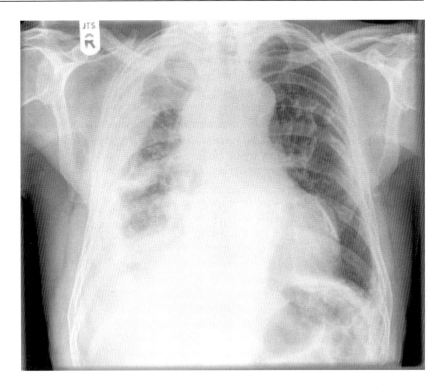

1   What is the most likely diagnosis?

☐ A   Asbestosis
☐ B   Squamous-cell carcinoma
☐ C   Pleural adenocarcinoma
☐ D   Mesothelioma
☐ E   Metastatic adenocarcinoma

2   Which of the investigations below is most likely to lead to a definitive diagnosis?

☐ A   Video-assisted thoracoscopic surgery (VATS) biopsy
☐ B   CT chest
☐ C   Chest drain and fluid sent for cytology
☐ D   CT-guided percutaneous needle biopsy
☐ E   Blind pleural biopsy with an Abraham's needle

Case 12

A 39-year-old lady from Zimbabwe presented to A&E with a 5-day history of increasing shortness of breath and dry cough. She had a 1-day history of sudden onset of sharp chest pain which was worse on coughing, movement and deep inspiration. She described having night sweats and a poor appetite for 2 months. Her weight had decreased by about 5 kg. She has a past medical history of genital herpes and depression. She is married and has two children who live in Zimbabwe. She moved to England 2 years ago and has not travelled since. She is a smoker of 20/day and drinks little alcohol.

On examination she looked unwell. Observations: temperature 38.3 °C, BP 108/72 mmHg, pulse 120 bpm, regular, respiratory rate 30/min. Auscultation of her chest revealed inspiratory crackles bibasally.

Investigations:

Hb	10.2 g/dL
WCC	9.4×10^9/L
Neutrophils	8.6×10^9/L
MCV	79 fL
Platelets	439×10^9/L
CRP	73 mg/L
Sodium	141 mmol/L
Potassium	4.2 mmol/L
Urea	5.0 mmol/L
Creatinine	75 µmol/L
Glucose	5.7 mmol/L

Blood gases on 80% oxygen:

pH	7.46
PCO_2	3.44 kPa
PO_2	19.77 kPa
Bicarbonate	17.6 mmol/L
Base excess	−3.5

Chest X-ray:

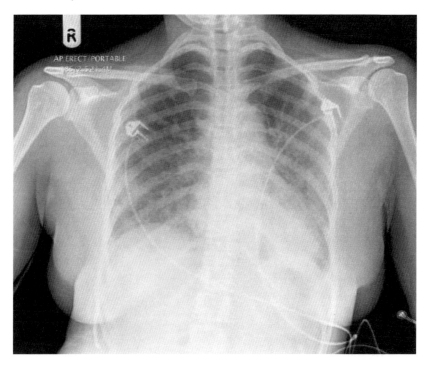

1 What is the most likely diagnosis?

- [ ] A *Legionella* pneumonia
- [ ] B *Pneumocystis carinii* pneumonia
- [ ] C Pulmonary embolus
- [ ] D Nocardiosis
- [ ] E CMV pneumonitis

2 Which investigation would be most helpful in establishing a diagnosis?

- [ ] A Bronchoscopy and transbronchial biopsy
- [ ] B CT pulmonary angiogram
- [ ] C Lung function tests and transfer factor
- [ ] D Indirect immunofluorescence of the bronchoalveolar lavage
- [ ] E Blood cultures

3   What is the most likely underlying cause?

☐ A   Lymphoma
☐ B   HIV
☐ C   Bronchiectasis
☐ D   Sarcoid
☐ E   Common variable immunodeficiency

4   What treatment should be started?

☐ A   Intravenous cephalosporin and clarithromycin
☐ B   Anticoagulation with warfarin
☐ C   Prednisolone
☐ D   Intravenous ganciclovir
☐ E   Intravenous high-dose co-trimoxazole ± steroids

Case 13

A 55-year-old woman presented with a 6-month history of recurrent chest infections. She had had a few episodes of wheeze and haemoptysis in the last few weeks. She also noticed intermittent hot flushes, which her GP had put down to the menopause. These could occur at any time but on occasions were precipitated by alcohol. She had no significant past medical history and she had never smoked.

On examination: she was anxious; examination of her chest revealed reduced expansion of the right upper zone; cardiovascular examination revealed a pansystolic murmur.

Blood results were unremarkable.

Chest X-ray:

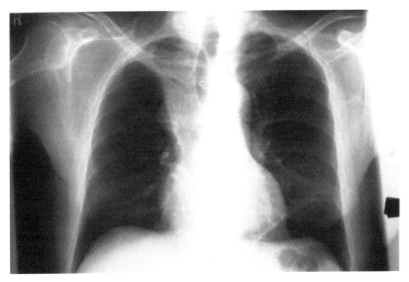

Image courtesy of Dr N Hughes, Frimley Park Hospital, Surrey

1 What two investigations would help you make a diagnosis?

- ☐ A Arterial blood gases
- ☐ B Spirometry
- ☐ C Urinary 5-hydroxyindoleacetic acid
- ☐ D Urinary catecholamines
- ☐ E Bronchoscopy and biopsy
- ☐ F Transfer factor
- ☐ G Methacholine challenge test
- ☐ H Bronchoscopy and bronchoalveolar lavage

2   What is the most likely diagnosis?

- [ ] A   Lymphoma
- [ ] B   Phaeochromocytoma
- [ ] C   Bronchial carcinoid
- [ ] D   Late-onset asthma
- [ ] E   Bronchiectasis

3   What is the treatment of choice?

- [ ] A   Surgery
- [ ] B   Steroid inhaler
- [ ] C   Intravenous antibiotics
- [ ] D   CHOP chemotherapy
- [ ] E   α-Adrenergic blockade, eg phenoxybenzamine

4   What does the chest X-ray show?

- [ ] A   Right upper lobe consolidation
- [ ] B   Right pleural effusion
- [ ] C   Right upper lobe calcification
- [ ] D   Right upper lobe collapse
- [ ] E   Right lower lobe collapse

Case 14

A 30-year-old man from London with no significant past medical history went on holiday to Peru to climb the Inca Trail. He is a non-smoker. After climbing above 3500 m he developed a headache, associated with nausea and vomiting. He also felt tired and complained of insomnia.

His respiratory rate was 22/min and his pulse was 90 bpm. Physical examination was unremarkable. No investigations are available as the nearest hospital is over 100 km away.

1   What is the most likely diagnosis?

- [ ] A   Exhaustion
- [ ] B   Hangover
- [ ] C   Migraine
- [ ] D   Acute mountain sickness
- [ ] E   Hypothermia

2   Which drug may have helped to prevent his symptoms?

- [ ] A   Aspirin
- [ ] B   Diazepam
- [ ] C   Furosemide
- [ ] D   Acetazolamide
- [ ] E   Propranolol

That night it was noticed that he was disorientated and walking with a broad-based gait and by the following morning he was drowsy and incoherent.

3   What is the most likely cause?

- [ ] A   High-altitude pulmonary oedema
- [ ] B   Cerebral haemorrhage
- [ ] C   Meningococcal septicaemia
- [ ] D   Cerebellar infarction
- [ ] E   High-altitude cerebral oedema

4   How would you treat this man?

- [ ] A   Immediate transfer down the mountain
- [ ] B   Aspirin
- [ ] C   Immediate antibiotics
- [ ] D   Acetazolamide and continue ascent
- [ ] E   Dexamethasone and continue ascent

Case 15

A 32-year-old man presents with recurrent chest infections productive of copious amounts of green purulent sputum. He had recurrent ear infections as a child. He is a smoker of 20/day and is married with no children.

On examination he is clubbed. Auscultation of his chest reveals coarse bibasal crackles and an expiratory wheeze. Heart sounds are normal. Abdominal examination is unremarkable except for a scar in the left iliac fossa.

Chest X-ray:

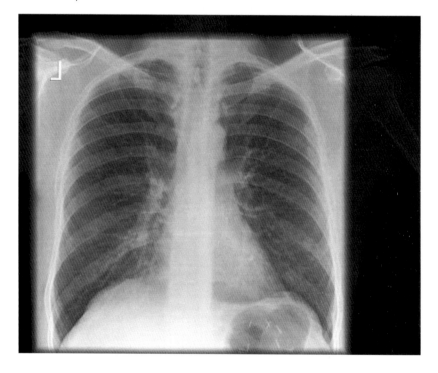

1   What is the cause of his recurrent chest infections?

- [ ] A   Asthma
- [ ] B   Allergic bronchopulmonary aspergillosis
- [ ] C   Bronchial obstruction
- [ ] D   Tuberculosis
- [ ] E   Bronchiectasis

2   Which investigation would you do to diagnose this?

- ☐ A   Histamine challenge test
- ☐ B   CT chest
- ☐ C   High-resolution CT chest
- ☐ D   *Aspergillus* precipitins
- ☐ E   Sputum culture

3   What is the complete diagnosis?

- ☐ A   Kartagener's syndrome
- ☐ B   Cystic fibrosis
- ☐ C   Young's syndrome
- ☐ D   Panhypogammaglobulinaemia
- ☐ E α_1-Antitrypsin deficiency

4   How would you confirm the diagnosis?

- ☐ A   Sweat test
- ☐ B α_1-Antitrypsin level
- ☐ C   Ciliary electron microscopy
- ☐ D   Serum immunoglobulins
- ☐ E   Testing nasal potential differences

Case 16

A 56-year-old man is referred to Outpatients with a 2-year history of increasing breathlessness and deteriorating exercise tolerance. He has a cough but is unable to produce any sputum. He complains of always feeling tired and has recently been asking his wife to help him look after his pigeons, which he has been racing for many years. He had lost about 1 stone in the last year. He has no history of recent foreign travel, except to France. He has a past medical history of asthma as a child. He has always worked in a bank. He is an ex-smoker and drinks minimal amounts of alcohol.

On examination he is not clubbed. On auscultation of his chest, he has fine inspiratory crackles.

ABGs on air:

pH	7.36
PO_2	7.4 kPa
PCO_2	4.7 kPa

Lung function tests:

FEV_1	70% predicted
FVC	64 % predicted
K_{CO}	53% predicted
T_{LCO}	55% predicted

Chest X-ray:

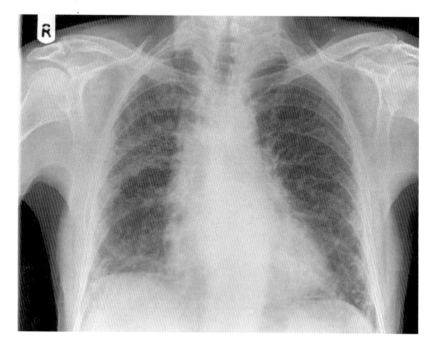

1   What is the most likely diagnosis?

☐ A   Cryptogenic fibrosing alveolitis (CFA)
☐ B   Extrinsic allergic alveolitis (EAA)
☐ C   Sarcoidosis
☐ D   Bronchopulmonary aspergillosis
☐ E   Psittacosis

2   Which of the following would help make a diagnosis?

☐ A   Serum ACE
☐ B   Avian serum precipitins
☐ C   *Aspergillus fumigatus* precipitins
☐ D   Blood cultures
☐ E   Bronchoscopy

Case 17

A 90-year-old man was referred to the clinic with a history of progressive shortness of breath and dry cough. Eighteen months ago he was able to complete a full round of golf. He stopped playing as he is now breathless after walking 200 m. He had been a heavy smoker all his life. He has no known asbestos exposure.

On examination he is breathless at rest. He has a photosensitive rash on his face and neck. He is clubbed. His pulse is irregularly irregular. Auscultation of his chest reveals fine inspiratory crackles bibasally.

Investigations:

		Blood gases on 30% oxygen:	
Hb	12.1 g/dL	pH	7.46
WCC	9.2×10^9/L	PCO_2	4.68 kPa
Neutrophils	6.1×10^9/L	PO_2	8.8 kPa
Platelets	203×10^9/L	Bicarbonate	25.4 mmol/L
TSH	7.1 mU/L		

Chest X-ray:

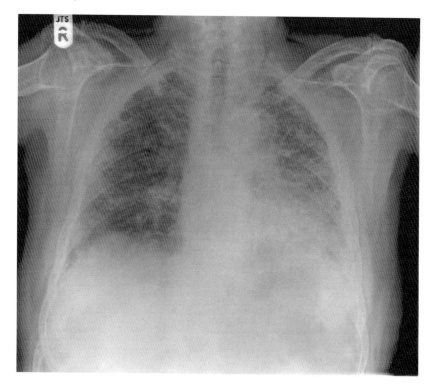

Spirometry:

FEV$_1$ 1.1 L (predicted 2.0–2.4 L)
FVC   2.0 L (predicted 3.2–3.8 L)
K$_{CO}$ 74% predicted

1   What is the likely cause of his breathlessness?

☐ A   COPD
☐ B   Pulmonary fibrosis
☐ C   Pulmonary oedema
☐ D   Bronchial alveolar carcinoma
☐ E   Lymphangioleiomyomatosis

2   What is the likely cause of the above diagnosis?

☐ A   Smoking
☐ B   Amiodarone
☐ C   Sarcoidosis
☐ D   Rheumatoid arthritis
☐ E   Pesticides

3   How would you confirm the diagnosis?

☐ A   High-resolution CT scan
☐ B   Echo
☐ C   Bronchoscopy and biopsy
☐ D   Open lung biopsy
☐ E   MRI chest

Case 18

A 25-year-old man presents with left-sided pleuritic chest pain. It had come on suddenly 3 days previously. Initially he thought it was secondary to his workout in the gym. However, since it did not improve and he noticed that he was slightly more breathless than usual, he went to A&E. He has no significant past medical history. He is a smoker of 20/day.

On examination he looked well. He was a tall thin man and was not short of breath at rest. Examination was unremarkable except for a clicking sound which was synchronous with the heart sounds.

Chest X-ray was unremarkable.

1   What is the diagnosis?

- ☐ A   Pericarditis
- ☐ B   Pleurisy
- ☐ C   Primary pneumothorax
- ☐ D   Secondary pneumothorax
- ☐ E   Mitral valve prolapse

2   Which of the following investigations may help with diagnosis?

- ☐ A   Repeat chest X-ray
- ☐ B   Echocardiogram
- ☐ C   Expiratory chest X-ray
- ☐ D   Lateral decubitus chest X-ray
- ☐ E   ECG

3   How would you manage this patient?

- ☐ A   Analgesia and discharge with follow-up in the clinic
- ☐ B   Non-steroidal anti-inflammatory drugs and admit patient
- ☐ C   Aspiration of chest
- ☐ D   Chest drain insertion
- ☐ E   Refer to Cardiology Department

Case 19

A 60-year-old man with known emphysema presented to A&E with sudden onset of severe left-sided pleuritic chest pain and shortness of breath. He is a smoker of 20/day.

On examination he looks unwell. He is pale and sweaty. BP 140/85 mmHg, pulse 120 bpm, respiratory rate 30/min, SaO_2 88% on air. He has reduced expansion and reduced breath sounds on the left side. Heart sounds were normal and abdominal examination unremarkable.

ABGs on air:
pH   7.41
PO_2 7.5 kPa
PCO_2 6.5 kPa

Chest X-ray:

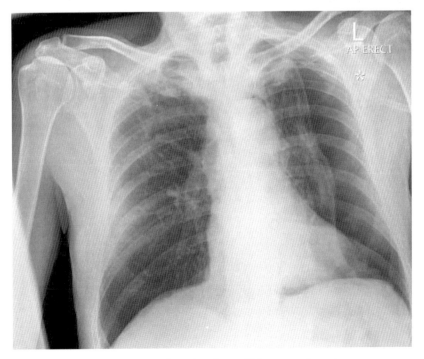

He is given 28% oxygen and analgesia and his saturations improve.

1 What would your immediate management of this patient be?

- ☐ A Chest aspiration
- ☐ B Insertion of an intercostal drain
- ☐ C Arrange an urgent CT scan of the chest
- ☐ D Refer to thoracic surgeons
- ☐ E Insertion of an intercostal tube and apply suction

After 4 days the lung is fully re-expanded. A chest drain has been inserted and is swinging and there is a persistent air leak despite suction (pressure $-20\,cmH_2O$).

2 What would you do?

- ☐ A Insert another chest drain
- ☐ B Increase suction pressure to $-30\,cmH_2O$
- ☐ C Refer to thoracic surgeons
- ☐ D Arrange a CT scan of the chest
- ☐ E Wait another 4 days

Case 20

A 31-year-old asthmatic woman was seen in Respiratory Outpatients. She said she had been generally well although she had not been sleeping well at night due to coughing. She had also noticed that when playing tennis she was getting wheezy and requiring her salbutamol inhaler more frequently – at least four times a week. She was taking budesonide 200 micrograms two puffs twice a day. She had no significant past medical history. She smoked 10 cigarettes a day and had done so for 2 years.

Auscultation of her chest revealed a mild expiratory wheeze. Examination was otherwise unremarkable.

PEF	80% predicted
FEV$_1$	85% predicted
FVC	90% predicted

1 How would you treat this patient?

- ☐ A Increase budesonide
- ☐ B Add an inhaled long-acting β$_2$-agonist
- ☐ C Give a course of oral prednisolone
- ☐ D Add aminophylline
- ☐ E Start regular salbutamol inhaler

Her symptoms improve and she goes back to playing regular tennis without a problem. Three months later she was feeling so much better she decided not to renew her prescription for her inhalers.

Two weeks following this she developed a chest infection and became acutely short of breath. On examination she is unable to speak full sentences. Respiratory rate 30/min, pulse 115 bpm, BP 100/60 mmHg.

Auscultation of her chest reveals an expiratory wheeze throughout.

PEFR 50 L/min

ABGs on air:

pH	7.45
PCO$_2$	4.06 kPa
PO$_2$	12 kPa
Bicarbonate	21.5 mmol/L

2   **Which of the following would be the best initial management for this patient?**

☐   A   High-flow oxygen, oral/intravenous steroid, salbutamol and ipratropium bromide nebuliser

☐   B   60% oxygen, oral/intravenous steroid, salbutamol and ipratropium bromide nebulisers and intravenous magnesium

☐   C   60% oxygen, oral/intravenous steroids, salbutamol and ipratropium bromide nebulisers and leukotriene receptor antagonist

☐   D   High-flow oxygen, salbutamol and ipratropium bromide nebulisers and intravenous magnesium

☐   E   High-flow oxygen, intravenous/oral steroids, ipratropium bromide nebuliser and intravenous aminophylline

She does not improve with treatment. Her chest examination now reveals quiet breath sounds. Repeat arterial blood gases on oxygen show:

pH	7.33
P_{CO_2}	6.5 kPa
P_{O_2}	12 kPa
Bicarbonate	25.1 mmol/L

3   **What would you do next?**

☐   A   Give more regular nebulisers
☐   B   Start non-invasive ventilation
☐   C   Refer to ICU for intubation
☐   D   Trial of heliox
☐   E   Give intravenous antibiotics

Case 21

A 77-year-old lady was referred to Respiratory Outpatients with increasing shortness of breath.

Chest X-ray:

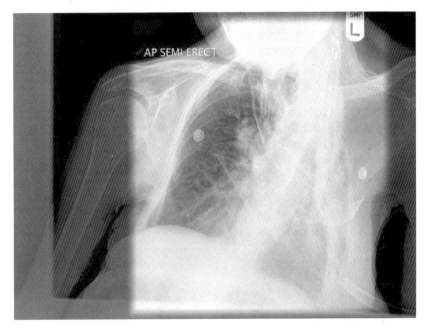

1   What operation has she had?

- ☐ A   Left pneumonectomy
- ☐ B   Phrenic crush
- ☐ C   Thoracoplasty
- ☐ D   Left upper lobectomy
- ☐ E   Plombage

2   What was the operation for?

- ☐ A   Small-cell lung cancer
- ☐ B   Squamous-cell lung cancer
- ☐ C   Adenocarcinoma
- ☐ D   Tuberculosis
- ☐ E   Recurrent pneumothoraces

Case 22

A 69-year-old gentleman was taken to A&E with a reduced GCS score. No history was available from the patient. The ambulance crew said the call was put out by his wife as he had become increasingly short of breath. When they arrived he had looked breathless and cyanosed. He had denied any chest pain.

On examination he has a GCS score of 10 (M5, V2, E3), respiratory rate 10/min, BP 130/70 mmHg, pulse 120 bpm, temperature 36.9 °C, SaO_2 94% on oxygen. Auscultation of his chest revealed an expiratory wheeze throughout.

Heart sounds were normal and abdominal examination unremarkable. There was no obvious focal neurological abnormality and both plantars showed a flexor response.

Investigations:

Hb	17.3 g/dL
WCC	8.2×10^9/L
MCV	84 fL
Platelets	400×10^9/L
CRP	21 mg/L

Renal function and liver function tests were unremarkable.
ECG – sinus tachycardia.
Chest X-ray – hyperinflated lung fields with low flattened diaphragms and there was no evidence of a pneumothorax.

In his notes you find a flow-volume curve from a year ago – see below:

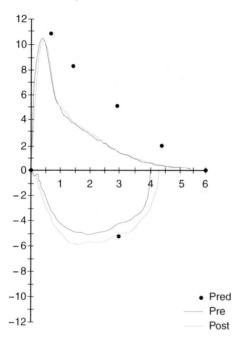

ABGs on high-flow oxygen:

pH	7.29
PCO₂	10.91 kPa
PO₂	12.39 kPa
Bicarbonate	40.6 mmol/L
Base excess	10.4

1   What does the arterial blood gas analysis show?

- [ ] A   Mixed respiratory and metabolic acidosis
- [ ] B   Acute respiratory acidosis
- [ ] C   Metabolic acidosis
- [ ] D   Acute on chronic respiratory acidosis
- [ ] E   Metabolic acidosis

2   What would your immediate management of this patient be?

- [ ] A Call anaesthetists for intubation
- [ ] B Start non-invasive ventilation
- [ ] C Hydrocortisone 100 mg intravenously
- [ ] D Salbutamol 2.5 mg via nebuliser
- [ ] E Reduce inspired oxygen concentration to 28% and repeat arterial blood gases

3   What does the flow-volume curve show?

- [ ] A Obstructive airways disease
- [ ] B A fixed extrathoracic airways disease obstruction
- [ ] C A variable extrathoracic airway disease obstruction
- [ ] D Restrictive lung disease
- [ ] E Intrathoracic airways obstruction

Case 23

A 72-year-old gentleman was referred to Respiratory Outpatients with a 2-month history of increasing shortness of breath and cough. Over the last few weeks he had coughed up a few streaks of blood. He has also noticed difficulty getting up from a chair. His wife noticed he had lost some weight but was unsure of the amount. He was taking regular inhalers.

On examination he was clubbed. Auscultation of his chest revealed reduced expansion and breath sounds on the left. Heart sounds were normal. He had 2-cm hepatomegaly. He had reduced power (4/5) on hip flexion bilaterally and generally reduced tendon reflexes. Plantars both showed a flexor response; proprioception and sensation were normal.

Investigations:

Hb	10.9 g/dL
WCC	12.2 × 10^9/L
MCV	79 fL
Platelets	491 × 10^9/L
ESR	58 mm/h
Sodium	126 mmol/L
Potassium	3.6 mmol/L
Urea	5.9 mmol/L
Creatinine	125 µmol/L
Bilirubin	49 µmol/L
AST	120 U/L
ALP	441 U/L
Albumin	32 g/L
Calcium	2.58 mmol/L
Phosphate	0.81 mmol/L

Chest X-ray:

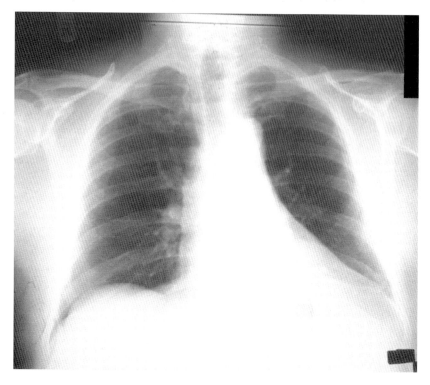

1   What does the chest X-ray show?

☐ A   Left lower lobe consolidation
☐ B   Left lower lobe collapse
☐ C   Lingular consolidation
☐ D   Left upper lobe collapse
☐ E   Small apical pneumothorax

2   Which investigations would you organise next to aid diagnosis and treatment?

☐ A   Bone scan and bronchoscopy
☐ B   CT brain and liver ultrasound
☐ C   Bronchoscopy and parathyroid hormone level
☐ D   MRI chest and bone scan
☐ E   CT chest/upper abdomen and bronchoscopy

3   What is the most likely underlying diagnosis?

☐ A   Adenocarcinoma of the lung
☐ B   Squamous carcinoma of the lung
☐ C   Small-cell carcinoma of the lung
☐ D   Mesothelioma
☐ E   Bronchial alveolar carcinoma

4   How would you treat this patient?

☐ A   Radiotherapy
☐ B   Lobectomy
☐ C   Pneumonectomy
☐ D   Chemotherapy
☐ E   Palliative care

5   What is the value of the corrected calcium?

☐ A   2.70 mmol/L
☐ B   2.74 mmol/L
☐ C   2.42 mmol/L
☐ D   2.40 mmol/L
☐ E   2.58 mmol/L

Case 24

A 45-year-old man presented to his GP with a gradual onset of shortness of breath and increasing difficulty swallowing.

Chest X-ray:

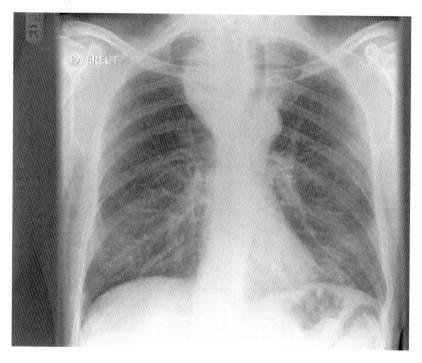

Flow-volume loop

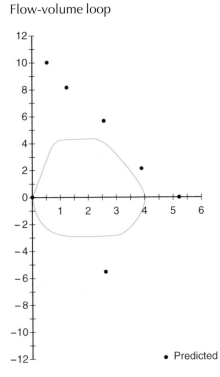

• Predicted

1   **What does the flow-volume loop show?**

- ☐ A   Fixed extrathoracic airflow obstruction
- ☐ B   Variable extrathoracic airflow obstruction
- ☐ C   Intrathoracic airflow obstruction
- ☐ D   Restrictive lung disease
- ☐ E   Obstructive lung disease

2   **What is the underlying cause?**

- ☐ A   Tracheal stenosis
- ☐ B   Chronic obstructive airways disease
- ☐ C   Vocal cord paralysis
- ☐ D   Idiopathic pulmonary fibrosis
- ☐ E   Goitre

Case 25

A 31-year-old lady presented to Respiratory Outpatients with a 3-year history of increasing shortness of breath and cough. She had required numerous courses of antibiotics in the last few years. She was a smoker of 5/day for about 5 years.

Respiratory examination revealed a hyperinflated chest and a mild wheeze throughout.

Lung function tests:

FEV_1	50% predicted
FVC	80% predicted
TLCO	68% predicted
KCO	71% predicted
RV:TLC	Increased

1 Which investigation would help make a diagnosis?

- ☐ A Histamine challenge test
- ☐ B Sweat test
- ☐ C Serum α_1-antitrypsin
- ☐ D Reversibility testing
- ☐ E High-resolution CT

2 What is the diagnosis?

- ☐ A Chronic obstructive pulmonary disease
- ☐ B Asthma
- ☐ C Cystic fibrosis
- ☐ D Bronchiectasis
- ☐ E α_1-Antitrypsin deficiency

Case 26

A 64-year-old gentleman was referred to the clinic with insomnia. He complained of falling asleep during the day and having an early morning headache. He had a past medical history of a cholecystectomy and gout. He took no other regular medication.

Examination was unremarkable.

Weight	120 kg
Height	175 cm
Hb	16.1 g/dL
WCC	6.4 × 10⁹/L
MCV	101 fL
Platelets	94 × 10⁹/L
TSH	1.2 mU/L

1   Which two of the following investigations would you arrange to aid diagnosis?

  A   Measurement of saturations on exertion
  B   Arterial blood gases
  C   Epworth score
  D   Echocardiogram
  E   Chest X-ray
  F   High-resolution CT chest
  G   Lung function tests and gas transfer
  H   Sleep studies
  I   Body plethysmography
  J   Six-minute walking test

2   What would your initial management of this patient be?

  A   Refer for non-invasive ventilation
  B   Diuretics
  C   Advise to lose weight
  D   Refer to ENT surgeons
  E   Doxapram

3   What underlying cause should be considered in this patient?

  A   Acromegaly
  B   Alcohol excess
  C   Hypothyroidism
  D   Cushing's disease
  E   Enlarged tonsils

Case 27

An 18-year-old woman presents with increasing shortness of breath. She has a past history of recurrent chest infections.

Look at the photograph of her fingers and her chest X-ray below:

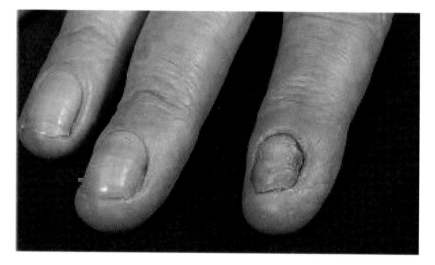

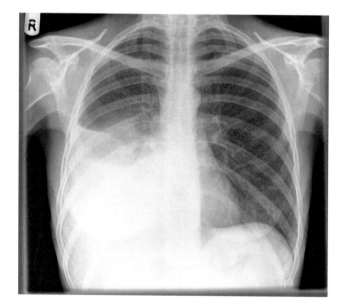

Sputum - mucopurulent

Pleural fluid:
Appearance   Clear
Protein   35 g/L
WCC   2440 (80% lymphocytes)

1   What is the most likely diagnosis?

☐ A   Cystic fibrosis
☐ B   Yellow-nail syndrome
☐ C   Filariasis
☐ D   Meigs' syndrome
☐ E   Tuberculosis

Case 28

A 25-year-old gentleman is brought into A&E following a road traffic accident in which he was thrown off his motorbike. He is complaining of pain in his chest and upper abdomen which radiates to his back and left shoulder. He was previously fit and well.

On examination he looks unwell. BP 90/55 mmHg, pulse 130 bpm. He is bruised and tender over his anterior chest wall. Auscultation of his chest reveals quiet breath sounds at the left base.

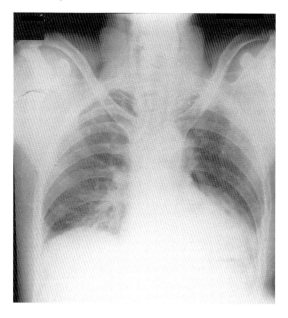

A diagnostic pleural tap is performed under ultra sound guidance.

Pleural fluid:
Protein	45 g/L
Amylase	240 U/L
Serum amylase	190 U/L

1   What is the diagnosis?

- [ ] A   Oesophageal rupture
- [ ] B   Pancreatitis
- [ ] C   Rib fractures and haemothorax
- [ ] D   Chylothorax
- [ ] E   Aortic dissection

Case 29

A 36-year-old man presents with increasing shortness of breath and a cough which is worse at night. He has no significant past medical history. He has never smoked. He works as a car mechanic, restoring run-down cars.

Examination is unremarkable.

FEV$_1$ 70% of normal
FVC   85% of normal
PEFR   450 L/min

Histamine challenge test:
20% fall in FEV$_1$ with 2 μmol histamine (normal > 4 μmol)

1   What is the most likely diagnosis?

☐ A   Carbon monoxide poisoning
☐ B   Occupational asthma
☐ C   Silicosis
☐ D   Extrinsic allergic alveolitis
☐ E   Hyper-reactive bronchial tree

Case 30

A 34-year-old HIV-positive man presented to hospital complaining of increasing shortness of breath and cough. He had noticed his vision was slightly worse over the last few weeks. He had a prolonged admission 4 months previously with a chest complaint. He was taking prophylactic co-trimoxazole. He smoked 20 cigarettes a day.

On examination he looked unwell. Pulse was 110 bpm, respiratory rate 28/min, BP 95/65 mmHg and saturations 91% on air. Auscultation of his chest revealed fine crackles bilaterally.

The chest X-ray shows reticular shadowing throughout both lung fields.

Bloods:

Hb	9.4 g/dL
WCC	3.2×10^9/L
MCV	84 fL
Platelets	511×10^9/L

CD4 count 10/mm^3

Sodium	139 mmol/L
Potassium	4.2 mmol/L
Urea	6.1 mmol/L
Creatinine	111 μmol/L
Bilirubin	52 μmol/L
AST	113 U/L
ALP	121 U/L
Albumin	34 U/L

TLCO   110% predicted

1   What is the likely diagnosis?

- [ ] A   *Pneumocystis carinii* pneumonia
- [ ] B   CMV pneumonitis
- [ ] C   *Nocardia* infection
- [ ] D   Tuberculosis
- [ ] E   Streptococcal pneumonia

2   How would you treat this patient?

- [ ]   A   Intravenous ganciclovir
- [ ]   B   High-dose intravenous co-trimoxazole
- [ ]   C   Quadruple anti-tuberculous chemotherapy (rifampicin, isoniazid, ethambutol and pyrazinamide)
- [ ]   D   Intravenous aciclovir
- [ ]   E   An intravenous cephalosporin

Case 31

A 16-year-old boy presents with a persistent cough productive of brown/ green sputum. He occasionally produces a small amount of blood. His mother said he had always suffered from chest infections, requiring numerous courses of antibiotics. He also complained of offensive-smelling stools which were difficult to flush.

On examination he looked small for his age. Auscultation of his chest revealed bibasal coarse crackles.

Investigations:

Hb	11.2 g/dL
WBC	10.7×10^9/L
MCV	91 fL
Platelets	511×10^9/L
Sodium	139 mmol/L
Potassium	3.9 mmol/L
Urea	5.3 mmol/L
Creatinine	99 μmol/L
Bilirubin	18 μmol/L
AST	34 U/L
ALP	93 U/L
Albumin	39 g/L
Total protein	50 g/L

Chest X-ray:

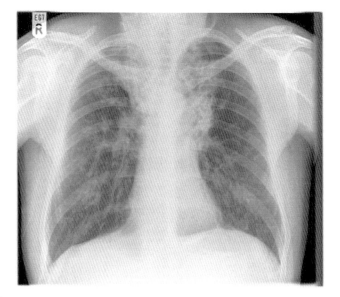

1 What is the diagnosis?

- [ ] A Cystic fibrosis
- [ ] B Kartagener's syndrome
- [ ] C Young's syndrome
- [ ] D X-linked hypogammaglobulinaemia
- [ ] E Primary ciliary dyskinesia

2 How would you make a diagnosis?

- [ ] A Sweat test
- [ ] B Measure immunoglobulins
- [ ] C Electron microscopy of cilia
- [ ] D High-resolution CT scan
- [ ] E Full lung function tests

Case 32

A 54-year-old man presented with increasing shortness of breath and orthopnoea. He had noticed these symptoms over the last few years but only went to his GP after he had had a severe episode of breathlessness when he went wading in the sea on holiday. On further enquiry he had also become aware of morning headaches and an increasing tendency to fall asleep during the day.

On examination he looked well. Auscultation of his chest revealed reduced breath sounds and percussion note bibasally.

Investigations:

Hb	17.7 g/dL
WCC	12.3 × 10^9/L
PCV	0.51
Platelets	289 × 10^9/L

	Erect (% predicted)	Supine (% predicted)
Residual volume	105%	
Total lung capacity	80%	
Vital capacity	75%	50%
T$_{LCO}$	70%	
K$_{CO}$	95%	

1   Which of the flowing is the least useful investigation?

- [ ] A   Chest X-ray
- [ ] B   Arterial blood gases
- [ ] C   Ultrasound screening of the diaphragm (SNIF test)
- [ ] D   Echocardiogram
- [ ] E   Gas transfer and transfer coefficient

2   What is the most likely diagnosis?

- [ ] A   Obstructive sleep apnoea
- [ ] B   Nocturnal asthma
- [ ] C   Bilateral diaphragmatic weakness
- [ ] D   Left ventricular failure
- [ ] E   Multiple sclerosis

ANSWERS

Chapter One   Answers

Case 1

1   D   Pericarditis

His ECG shows classic features of acute pericarditis, with a sinus tachycardia, widespread concave ST elevation, and PR depression. In acute pericarditis PR depression is frequently seen; it is almost never seen in acute ischaemia. It is not unusual to get a troponin rise in acute pericarditis. Misdiagnosis of such a case could lead to inappropriate thrombolysis with serious consequences. A fever is a common finding in acute pericarditis. Occasionally, pericarditis pain can radiate, mimicking angina. Most cases of acute pericarditis are self-limiting and resolve in a few weeks with conservative treatment. Non-steroidal anti-inflammatory drugs (NSAIDs) are the first-line therapy of choice in acute pericarditis.

Case 2

1   E   Admit him, treat him as if he had acute coronary syndrome and repeat his troponin in 12 hours

Patients are notoriously unreliable with recalling their history; troponin should be measured 12 hours after admission to hospital to exclude myocardial damage. If in doubt, any patient with a history of chest pain and labile ECG changes should be treated initially as if they had acute coronary syndrome. In this case, if the troponin is positive in 12 hours, then the patient should be referred for inpatient angiography.

Case 3

1   C   Have an AICD inserted prior to discharge

An out-of-hospital cardiac arrest is a primary indication for the insertion of an AICD if the ejection fraction is less than 30%, irrespective of the aetiology, as supported by data from the MADIT I trial.[1]

---

[1] Moss AJ, Hall WJ, Cannom DS, Daubert JP, Higgins SL, Klein H, Levine JH, Saksena S, Waldo AL, Wilber D, Brown MW and Heo M. (MADIT Investigators). 1996. Improved survival with an implanted defibrillator in patients with coronary disease at high risk of ventricular arrhythmias. *New England Journal of Medicine* 335, 1933–1940.

Case 4

1   D   Pulmonary stenosis and Noonan's syndrome

Noonan's syndrome is classically associated with pulmonary valve lesions, but occasionally can be associated with cardiomyopathies. This patient has pulmonary stenosis, with an ejection systolic murmur heard loudest over the left upper sternal edge, and normal pulse character and blood pressure. Noonan's syndrome patients classically have a webbed neck, pectus excavatum and cryptorchidism. Turner's syndrome patients look similar but Turner's produces a phenotypic female, is associated with coarctation of the aorta, bicuspid aortic valve and aortic dilatation.

Case 5

1   B   Brugada syndrome

Brugada syndrome is a cause of ventricular tachycardia and ventricular fibrillation; it is associated with right bundle branch block and ST elevation in the anterior pre-cordial leads. AICD insertion is the treatment of choice. Wolff–Parkinson–White syndrome is associated with a δ wave on the resting ECG. Jervell and Lange-Nielsen syndrome is associated with deafness and long QT syndrome, which predisposes to fatal ventricular arrhythmias, especially *torsades de pointes*.

Case 6

1   C   Situs inversus

The X-ray shows dextrocardia and a right-sided gastric bubble, consistent with situs inversus (see below). It is likely he has appendicitis (left-sided with situs inversus). Given the history of recurrent sinusitis, Kartagener's syndrome is a likely diagnosis but one cannot say this for sure by just looking at the chest X-ray.

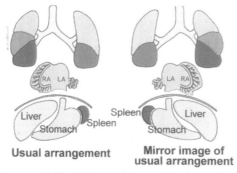

Image provided by Dr Ho, Royal Brompton Hospital, London

Case 7

1   **A**   Ensure he has an inpatient echocardiogram prior to discharge

The presentation and signs clearly point to a new diagnosis of aortic stenosis. Severe aortic stenosis with a history of blackouts carries a very high mortality if not treated. He must have an echocardiogram to confirm the clinical diagnosis and to assess the gradient and left ventricular function. If he has severe aortic stenosis he should be referred to the cardiologists as an inpatient. Exercise testing is contraindicated in severe aortic stenosis.

Case 8

1   **D**   Insertion of a temporary pacing wire to allow further diagnostic tests and management

There are few causes of sudden-onset complete heart block in a young fit patient like this. She has been in New England (where Lyme disease is endemic) and Lyme disease with acquired AV block is the most likely diagnosis. The rash is likely to be erythema chronicum migrans, which is the classic migratory rash seen in the initial phase of Lyme disease. A temporary pacing wire should be inserted to allow serological confirmation of the diagnosis and treatment with a course of appropriate antibiotics. The heart block nearly always resolves with appropriate treatment, usually within a week, after which the temporary pacing wire can be removed.

Case 9

1   **E**   Intravenous flecainide

She clearly has Wolff–Parkinson–White (WPW) syndrome, as evidenced by the short PR interval and δ wave on her resting ECG. Digoxin and verapamil must never be used in this condition as both can provoke fatal arrhythmias (VT/VF) in patients with WPW. Adenosine is contraindicated because of her asthma. DC cardioversion is only used as first choice in patients who are haemodynamically compromised.

Case 10

1   **C**   Ischaemic ventricular septal defect needing urgent intra-aortic balloon pump and referral for surgery

He clearly has an ischaemic ventricular septal defect (VSD), as demonstrated by the step-up in oxygen saturations in the pulmonary artery. These classically occur 3–5 days post-myocardial infarction. 90% of post-infarct VSDs are associated with a new murmur. Mortality is 90%

with medical treatment and 50% with surgical treatment. An intra-aortic balloon pump will help support his circulation while he gets to theatre.

Case 11

1   **E**   Administer thrombolysis, provided there are no contraindications (tPA and intravenous heparin)

She has had an anterior ST-elevation MI. She should be treated with thrombolysis in the first instance. Streptokinase is never given with intravenous heparin. In the trials to date aspirin and clopidogrel have only shown to be of benefit in non-ST-elevation MI; tPA has been shown to achieve better reperfusion in patients with an anterior MI and is always given with a 24-hour intravenous heparin infusion. Primary percutaneous intervention has been shown to be superior to administration of thrombolysis, provided patients can be transferred within 3 hours (PRAGUE-2[1] and DANAMI-2[2] trials). In the UK in most district general hospitals, administration of thrombolysis is still the treatment of first choice; however this could change with improved resources and facilities in the future. In the scenario presented here the patient is clearly going to take at least 3 hours to be transferred to the intervention centre, so they should be treated with thrombolysis in the first instance.

[1] http://www.medscape.com/viewarticle/442509
[2] http://www.danami-2.dk/Index.htm

Case 12

1   **C**   Peripartum cardiomyopathy

Peripartum cardiomyopathy by definition occurs between 1 month prior to delivery and up to 6 months post-partum and is a diagnosis of exclusion. There is no preceding history of a viral illness here, so a post-viral cardiomyopathy is unlikely, although one would of course check viral titres. Peripartum cardiomyopathy usually has a good prognosis, although it can recur in subsequent pregnancies. It is treated with angiotensin-converting enzyme (ACE) inhibitors and patients usually need formal anticoagulation. If it is diagnosed prior to delivery, then hydralazine is the drug of choice until the baby has been delivered, as ACE inhibitors can be harmful to the baby.

Case 13

1   **B**   *Torsades de pointes*

2   **B**   He has acquired long QT syndrome due to his neuroleptic medication

This is classic *torsades de pointes* (also called 'polymorphic ventricular tachycardia'), showing the well-described twisting morphology.

Long QT syndrome classically causes *torsades de pointes* and the most likely cause is his neuroleptic medication: this should be withdrawn and his long QT (QT 480ms, QTc 537ms) will resolve. Ischaemia should always be ruled out as a precipitating cause.

Case 14

1   **A**   His echocardiogram shows asymmetrical septal hypertrophy. The diagnosis is hypertrophic cardiomyopathy. He should be considered for an AICD insertion

He has hypertrophic cardiomyopathy and is at high risk of sudden death and should have an AICD inserted. Myomectomy is only indicated if there is a significant outflow tract gradient; this is normally now done medically by angiographic injection of the septal perforator arteries with alcohol to induce septal necrosis and thinning. An AICD is superior to amiodarone for the long-term prevention of sudden death; furthermore, AICD also has none of the toxicity associated with amiodarone.

Case 15

1   **D**   Her ECG shows sinus rhythm and left bundle branch block and she should be treated for pulmonary oedema and considered for CPAP if she does not respond to the initial treatment

She has a clinical presentation of acute pulmonary oedema due to left ventricular failure. She has not had any chest pain and there is no indication for giving thrombolysis. Her ECG shows classic left bundle branch block, which is often seen in long-standing hypertensive patients. Her history is clearly suggestive of worsening left ventricular failure with increasing breathlessness on exertion, orthopnoea and ankle swelling. Initially she should be treated by offloading her heart with intravenous GTN and/or diuretics. Failing this, non-invasive ventilation with CPAP can be of great benefit in the acute management of pulmonary oedema. She does not have cardiogenic shock, by definition, with this blood pressure. To interpret the left ventricular strain pattern seen with left bundle branch block as lateral ischaemia is an error.

Case 16

1   **D**   His ECG shows right bundle branch block; his murmur is likely to be due to pulmonary regurgitation. This can be associated with an increased risk of sudden death and he needs further investigation

Tetralogy of Fallot patients who have had corrective surgery are at an increased risk of developing late pulmonary regurgitation as a complication. This was previously thought to be a relatively benign condition, but it is now known that as the severity of the regurgitation worsens, the patients are at an increased risk of ventricular arrhythmias and sudden death. Patients with pulmonary regurgitation must be investigated further, with an echo at least. These patients should be referred to see a specialist in adult congenital heart disease if the severity of the pulmonary regurgitation is moderate or worse. Right bundle branch block can be a normal ECG finding; however, in this patient it is likely to be a result of previous cardiac surgery.

Case 17

1   **B**   He has mitral regurgitation and should have a transoesophageal echocardiogram (TOE) to define the anatomy better. If possible, the first choice of treatment should be mitral valve repair

His echocardiogram shows a colour jet extending into the left atrium, consistent with mitral regurgitation. Where possible, the mitral valve should always be repaired as first choice; this gives a better physiological result and if in the future re-do surgery is needed improves the chances of this being successful. In severe mitral regurgitation you should not wait until the left ventricle decompensates before referring a patient for surgery as this is too late; the patient should be referred as soon as possible.

Case 18

1   **B**   He has cardiogenic shock; if possible, a Swan–Ganz catheter should be inserted to optimise his haemodynamics. He should have an urgent echo (if available) and you should consider insertion of an intra-aortic balloon pump, transferring him urgently to an intervention centre provided you can get him stable enough

Cardiogenic shock post-MI carries a mortality of around 90% in patients managed medically. The SHOCK trial showed that cardiac intervention within the first 24 hours significantly reduces this mortality (to around 70%). An intra-aortic balloon pump (IABP), if available, will help stabilise the patient for transfer by improving perfusion of the coronary arteries in diastole. Administration of thrombolysis is not indicated, as there is no evidence of persistent ST elevation or pain. A Swan–Ganz catheter will help you manage him haemodynamically while you prepare/get him stable for transfer. The priority is to get an IABP inserted as soon as possible and the patient transferred for intervention as soon as is safe and practical.

Case 19

1   **C**   She has an inferior ST-elevation MI with complete heart block and should be given thrombolysis as soon as possible

Complete heart block is often seen with an inferior MI; this usually resolves within 2 weeks. Pacing is not necessary unless the patient is haemodynamically compromised. The faster thrombolysis is administered, the more likely this will resolve. Some people would insert a pacing sheath in A&E prior to giving thrombolysis so that if the patient were to require pacing this would be more straightforward and associated with fewer complications; this approach is reasonable provided it does not unduly delay administration of thrombolysis.

Case 20

1   **D**   Discuss his case with one of the cardiologists at his centre

Patients with complex adult congenital heart disease must always be discussed with an expert in this field promptly; they are always happy to give advice and will often accept these patients for further management. The circulation in these patients is often very complex and finely balanced and treating common cardiac problems in the usual way can have disastrous effects. Furthermore, these patients often need the expertise of cardiac anaesthetists who are experienced in dealing with these conditions, even for seemingly straightforward surgical procedures such as an appendicectomy. Flecainide should never be given to people with structural heart disease.

Case 21

1   **A**   Monomorphic ventricular tachycardia

2   **C**   Synchronised DC cardioversion

This is classic monomorphic VT: wide-complex regular tachycardia with concordance in the chest leads and extreme axis deviation; fusion and/or capture beats are often seen.

He has VT, which is compromising his blood pressure, and should be cardioverted urgently as he is at an increasing risk of having a cardiac arrest (VF) the longer this is left.

Case 22

1   **B**   She should be anticoagulated with warfarin, have her rate controlled with medication, have an echocardiogram and be brought back for an elective cardioversion in 6–8 weeks

She is not haemodynamically compromised by her AF and cardioversion carries an unacceptable risk of a thromboembolic event (such as a stroke). She has no prior history of AF and so an attempt to cardiovert her should be made. However, this should be done after she has been formally anticoagulated for 6–8 weeks. In the meantime, medication can be used to control her ventricular rate. If the patient is haemodynamically compromised then the risk of thromboembolism is outweighed and she should be urgently cardioverted. If available, the best alternative would be an urgent TOE to rule out thrombus in the left atrium, followed by cardioversion; these patients should have peri-procedure heparin cover and 6 weeks of formal anticoagulation post-cardioversion. Thromboembolic events as a result of AF cause 20% of stokes; patients with AF should be anticoagulated with warfarin (target INR 2–3) to prevent thromboembolic complications. Aspirin is inferior to warfarin and should be reserved for patients with contraindications to warfarin (such as those at a high risk of falls).

Case 23

1   D   Mitral stenosis

The ECG shows P mitrale (broad bifid P waves), which is consistent with left atrial dilatation. Rheumatic heart disease is still relatively common in the Third World. A percutaneous valvuloplasty can be considered to relieve symptoms if necessary but a TOE should be arranged first to assess suitability for this.

Case 24

1   C   Atrial myxoma

Fibroelastomas are small benign tumours, usually found on valves, which have a tendency to present as emboli. Her examination is normal so she clearly does not have AF. Myxomas are benign tumours treated by surgical excision.

Case 25

1   E   Stop warfarin 4 days before the operation; admit the patient the next day and put them on a full therapeutic dose of intravenous heparin. Stop the heparin 4 hours prior to the surgery, then restart it afterwards; keep the patient on heparin until they are back on warfarin and the desired INR is reached

Never stop a patient's warfarin without ensuring they have adequate intravenous heparin cover if they have a mechanical heart valve, especially if it is in the mitral position and/or it is a ball-and-cage type of valve. Prosthetic mitral valves, especially Starr–Edwards, are at high risk of developing thrombi, the consequences of which can be disastrous.

Case 26

1   **C**   Reassure the nurse that no anti-arrhythmics are necessary, but that an insulin sliding scale should be started

Apart from correction of electrolytes (if abnormal), pharmacological treatment of ectopics and bigeminy, in the acute phase post-MI, is not necessary. In some cases, prescription of anti-arrhythmic agents in this situation worsens mortality (CAST trial[1]). Strict control of blood sugars post-MI improves mortality (DIGAMI trial[2]) and an insulin sliding scale should be started in these patients.

[1] The Cardiac Arrhythmia Suppression Trial (CAST) Investigators. 1989. Effects of encainide and flecainide on mortality in a randomized trial of arrhythmia suppression after myocardial infarction. *New England Journal of Medicine*, 321, 406–412.
[2] Malmberg K, Ryden L, Hamsten A, Herlitz J, Waldenstrom A, Wedel H, Welin L. 1995. Randomized trial of insulin-glucose infusion followed by subcutaneous insulin treatment in diabetic patients with acute myocardial infarction (DIGAMI study): effects on mortality at 1 year. *Journal of the American College of Cardiology* 26, 56–65.

Case 27

1   **B**   Start non-invasive ventilation and arrange an urgent echocardiogram and cardiology review

He clearly has aortic regurgitation with pulmonary oedema, the most likely cause of which is endocarditis. Intra-aortic balloon pump insertion is contraindicated in aortic regurgitation. Non-invasive ventilation is excellent for the treatment of acute pulmonary oedema; an echo will confirm your clinical diagnosis. The cardiothoracic surgeons will need to be involved. It is likely that he will need an aortic valve replacement, the timing of which will be critical.

Case 28

1   **C**   Do a dipstick urinalysis and send off an MSU; consider antibiotics, depending on the result, and admit her for further investigation

There is no evidence that she has endocarditis. You need to exclude simple things first, such as a UTI, and you will need to investigate her anaemia, which could be due to an underlying malignancy. A transthoracic echocardiogram is the first-choice investigation in suspected endocarditis. The modified Duke criteria are useful in the diagnosis of endocarditis and should be used (this patient fulfills none of these criteria at present).

Case 29

1   **D**   Take blood cultures, start him on intravenous antibiotics for

endocarditis, ensure his anticoagulation is therapeutic and arrange a cardiology opinion as soon as possible

This is quite the opposite of the last case. Endocarditis early after a valve replacement is usually staphylococcal and carries a high mortality (up to 70%). These patients need aggressive treatment and antibiotics should be started without delay once blood cultures are taken. Cardiology input within either that or the next working day is essential, unless the patient is in any way unstable, in which case he should be discussed with the cardiologists on call. Although a transthoracic echo is helpful, a TOE is usually needed to fully assess a prosthetic valve.

Case 30

1   **C**   Tetralogy of Fallot

Tetralogy of Fallot consists of: perimembranous VSD (as evidenced by step-up in saturations at right ventricular (RV) level and high pressures), infundibular RVOT obstruction (as evidenced by normal pulmonary artery pressure in face of high RV pressure), RV hypertrophy and over-riding aorta. The worse the RVOT obstruction is, the worse the symptoms and prognosis are. This patient would need more imaging, starting with an echocardiogram, and referral to the paediatric cardiologists.

Case 31

1   **C**   Speak to the microbiologists and say you suspect an atypical organism (HACEK), and ask them to look for this and check whether your current therapy covers these organisms

This patient clearly has endocarditis. He has improved on antibiotics and has had a vegetation demonstrated on his echocardiogram. The fastidious organisms (HACEK: *Haemophilus* spp.; *Actinobacillus actinomycetemcomitans; Cardiobacterium hominis, Eikenella* spp. and *Kingella kingae*) do not grow with routine microbiology culture techniques. The microbiologists will not usually set up cultures to look for these organisms unless you ask them. The HACEK organisms cause around 10% of cases of endocarditis in patients with long-term valve replacements. Microbiology input is very important in any case of endocarditis and you should always liaise closely with them. Fungal endocarditis is unusual in an immunocompetent patient and often causes large vegetations. If a vegetation is clearly seen on transthoracic echocardiogram you do not necessarily need a TOE.

Case 32

E Friedreich's ataxia

Friedreich's ataxia presents with difficulty in walking from around age 12; it is associated with cerebellar ataxia, dysarthria, nystagmus and dysdiadochokinesis. It is associated with cardiomyopathy, which can cause cardiac failure.

Duchenne muscular dystrophy presents at a much younger age and few patients survive beyond the age of 20 years.

Case 33

1 D Take further blood cultures and organise another TOE

A lengthening PR interval is a sign of an aortic root abscess developing; these are not always seen on transthoracic echo and a TOE is the investigation of choice. Surgery is often necessary.

Case 34

1 A Pseudoxanthoma elasticum

The 'plucked chicken skin' appearance is classic of pseudoxanthoma elasticum, which is associated with abnormalities of the skin, eyes and blood vessels. It is associated with early-onset ischaemic heart and peripheral vascular disease. Angioid streaks are seen on funduscopy.

Case 35

1 D Percutaneous device closure

He has pulmonary hypertension with no evidence of an ASD or VSD. The most likely diagnosis in a young, otherwise fit patient like this is primary pulmonary hypertension. Intravenous epoprostenol (prostacyclin), sildenafil and diltiazem have all been shown to improve symptoms but have little effect on the ultimate prognosis. Cardiac transplantation is the only treatment that has been shown to improve survival. There is no evidence of an ASD or VSD, therefore no role for percutaneous device closure.

Case 36

1 B Atrial septal defect (ASD)

She has a step-up in her oxygen saturations, at the level of the right atrium; this is never normal. The diagnosis is an ASD. She will need a shunt calculation and further imaging with a TOE; depending on these results, she may benefit from a device closure.

Case 37

1   **D**   Start her on a β-blocker to control her heart rate

She has Waldenström's macroglobulinaemia and probably has cardiac amyloid as a result of this. Cardiac amyloid is predominantly seen in the AL type of amyloid, which is caused by Waldenström's macroglobulinaemia, myeloma and non-Hodgkin's lymphoma. Digoxin should be avoided in amyloid disease as the amyloid fibrils bind digoxin and significant toxicity can occur, even with low doses of digoxin. Systolic function is often normal in cardiac amyloid; a speckled appearance in the myocardium is typical of cardiac amyloid. The prognosis in cardiac amyloid is generally poor, with the exception of familial amyloidosis (which may respond to transplantation).

Case 38

1   **E**   He should be put an a nitrate infusion and have either a TOE or a CT chest with contrast

Clinically, he has an aortic dissection, as the dissection extends back into the coronary root it extends into the right coronary artery, causing inferior ischaemia. Acute aortic regurgitation is also often seen. A common misconception is that a wide mediastinum is always seen with dissection. This is usually only seen with traumatic aortic dissections. TOE or CT chest with contrast are the investigations of choice; an experienced operator should perform the TOE, ideally in a cardiothoracic centre. Blood pressure should be tightly regulated; usually labetalol is the first agent of choice but not in this case where the patient is asthmatic. Anticoagulation or thrombolysis of these patients can result in disaster.

Case 39

1   **E**   Switch his atenolol to bisoprolol and start him on ramipril

He has moderate LV dysfunction and should be titrated onto an ACE inhibitor up to the optimal dose. He should be switched to one of the β-blockers licensed for cardiac failure (such as carvedilol or bisoprolol) and the dose of this should be gradually titrated up every 2 weeks until the optimum dose is reached. There is now evidence that even patients with severe LV dysfunction benefit from β-blockers, provided they are not on intravenous inotropes or vasodilators (CAPRICORN and COPERNICUS trials). Spironolactone should only be used in patients with severe ventricular dysfunction (RALES trial). Clopidogrel in addition to aspirin is only used after a non-ST-elevation MI. His statin dose should be optimised.

Case 40

1   **D**   Start him on oral digoxin

He has fast AF on top of underlying left bundle branch block; this is often confused with VT by the inexperienced. Unlike VT, it is irregular and there is no concordance, caption or fusion beats. He should be started on oral digoxin to control his ventricular rate; an additional agent is often needed to achieve this (such as a β-blocker). He should be considered for formal anticoagulation and the standard investigation/management of AF.

Chapter Two   Answers

Case 1

1   **B**   *Legionella pneumophila*

2   **B**   Urinary *Legionella* antigen

Legionella has three epidemiological patterns:

- Outbreaks due to contaminated water-cooling systems, air-conditioning or showers. May be an occupational history or recent hotel holiday. Usually occurs in previously fit individuals. This man worked in a law firm and it is presumed this contains an air-conditioning system.
- Sporadic causes. Rare at extremes of age. Usually age 40–70. More common in men than in women. At-risk groups: smokers, chronic illness – especially chest disease, diabetes mellitus – and alcoholics.
- Outbreaks occurring in immunosuppressed individuals, eg those on corticosteroids.

The incubation period is 2–10 days and it typically presents with flu-like symptoms – fevers, malaise, myalgia and headaches; the patient later develops cough, breathlessness and confusion; 50% develop gastointestinal symptoms.

Investigations: hyponatraemia, lymphopenia, haematuria, proteinuria and hypoxia. Abnormal liver biochemistry (especially aminotransferases) and renal function occur in 50% of patients.

Diagnosis: the quickest way is to test for urinary *Legionella* antigen, and direct immunofluorescent staining of the organism in sputum, pleural fluid, or bronchial washings. Gram stain does not usually reveal an organism. Acute and convalescent serology – diagnosis is made on a fourfold rise in antibody titre to > 1:128. Convalescent serology should be taken between 8 and 12 weeks after onset, thus delaying diagnosis. Chest X-ray (CXR) usually shows lobar and then multilobar shadowing. Small pleural effusions may occur.

Treatment is with a macrolide. The other clue in this question is the lack of response to β-lactam antibiotics.

Case 2

1 **E** *Mycoplasma* pneumonia

2 **C** *Mycoplasma* serology
   D Cold agglutinins

Mycoplasma usually affects young individuals and occurs in epidemics every 3–4 years. Chest symptoms are usually preceded by non-specific symptoms such as malaise and headaches.

The CXR usually shows only one lobe to be involved; however, about 20% show bilateral pneumonia. There is often a discrepancy between X-ray appearances and the clinical condition of the patient.

Diagnosis is by *Mycoplasma* serology; cold agglutinins occur in 50%. The image shows erythema multiforme, which further supports the diagnosis. The blood results suggest a haemolytic anaemia with a reticulocytosis, hyperbilirubinaemia and elevated LDH; Autoimmune haemolytic anaemia (AIHA), when caused by cold agglutinins, is associated with *Mycoplasma* and can be diagnosed with a direct Coombs' test.

Extrapulmonary complications of *Mycoplasma* include:

- Cardiovascular – myocarditis and pericarditis
- Dermatological – erythema multiforme, Stevens–Johnson syndrome and non-specific rashes
- Gastrointestinal – hepatitis, pancreatitis, nausea, vomiting, anorexia and transient abdominal pain
- Neurological – meningoencephalitis, meningitis, ascending paralysis transient myelitis, cranial nerve palsies, peripheral neuropathy
- Haematological – cold autoimmune haemolytic anaemia, thrombocytopenia
- Renal – glomerulonephritis
- Others – arthralgia, arthritis, bullous myringitis.

Treatment: a macrolide.

Causes of erythema multiforme:

- Infections – herpes simplex virus (most common cause), orf, HBV, HIV, EBV, mumps (paramyxovirus), *Mycoplasma*, psittacosis, rickettsiae, *Streptococcus*, typhoid, diphtheria
- Drug reactions – barbiturates, penicillin, sulphonamides, phenytoin
- Connective tissue disease – SLE
- Vasculitis – polyarteritis nodosa, Wegener's granulomatosis
- Others – underlying malignancy, sarcoidosis, rheumatoid arthritis, ulcerative colitis.

Case 3

1   **A**   Silicosis

2   **C**   Mixed respiratory and metabolic acidosis

3   **B**   Insert a left-sided chest drain

Silicosis is a fibrotic lung disease associated with inhalation of silica (silicon dioxide), which is highly fibrogenic. It is usually seen in quarrying and mining tunnelling occupations and in sandblasters, ceramic workers, pottery workers and in stonemasons if the dust generated contains quartz.

Silicosis may present as an acute illness following very heavy exposure or run a more chronic course as in this patient. Diagnosis is made on history of exposure and chest X-ray changes. The chest X-ray may show hilar eggshell calcification (pathognomonic of silicosis), as in the chest X-ray shown, with or without upper zone fibrosis.

This man also has an element of chronic obstructive pulmonary disease (COPD) – mixed obstructive and restrictive spirometry (FEV_1 more markedly reduced than FVC) and a history of smoking. He later presents with an exacerbation, made worse by his underlying silicosis, with a mixed respiratory and metabolic acidosis. He is commenced on a trial of non-invasive ventilation (NIV) and initially does well. He later desaturates as he develops a pneumothorax. The treatment of choice in any ventilated patient with a pneumothorax is insertion of a chest drain. If the patient had a tension pneumothorax, a chest drain should be inserted after initial decompression with a cannula.

Case 4

1   **D**   Pulmonary embolism (PE)

2   **D**   Alteplase

This lady has had a massive pulmonary embolus. She presented with shortness of breath and tachypnoea. Her arterial blood gases show she has type I respiratory failure; note the low CO_2 – common in PE.

The CT scan shows large filling defects in the left and right main pulmonary arteries.

The aim of this question is to ensure the candidate is aware of the British Thoracic Society guidelines on the treatment of massive PE.[1] The

[1] British Thoracic Society Standards of Care Committee, Pulmonary Embolism Guidelines Development Group. 2003. British Thoracic Society guidelines for the management of suspected acute pulmonary embolism. *Thorax*, 58, 470–484. http://www.brit-thoracic.org.uk/index.asp

guidelines state that if a PE is severe enough to cause circulatory collapse, thrombolysis should be given as early as possible. The current guidelines recommend alteplase as the thrombolytic agent of choice as it can be given to the hypotensive patient, as in this example.

Case 5

1   **C**   Aspiration pneumonia

This is aspiration pneumonia. This lady is an alcoholic (thrombocytopenia, macrocytosis, raised INR and abnormal liver function tests, in particular the γGT). She has consumed too much alcohol on Christmas Day, fallen (note creatine kinase) and aspirated. The chest X-ray shows a right lower lobe pneumonia consistent with an aspiration pneumonia.

Case 6

1   **D**   Sarcoidosis

2   **C**   Bronchoscopy and transbronchial biopsies

The most likely diagnosis is sarcoidosis. This is a relatively young patient with breathlessness, dry eyes, fatigue, night sweats and polyuria. He has a normocytic anaemia, a raised ESR and slightly deranged liver function tests.

Sarcoid is a multisystem granulomatous disorder with a number of different presentations. It usually presents in the under-forties, and is more common in women.

The diagnosis is suggested from a chest X-ray and high-resolution CT. Pulmonary involvement can be classified according to the radiographic stage of the disease as below:

Stage 1: Bihilar adenopathy
Stage 2: Bihilar adenopathy and interstitial infiltrates
Stage 3: Interstitial disease with shrinking hilar nodes
Stage 4: Advanced fibrosis

Transbronchial biopsy is the investigation with the highest yield as positive results are seen in 90% of patients with pulmonary sarcoidosis. Endobronchial biopsies are also useful but less sensitive.

Serum ACE is not specific as raised levels are also seen in pulmonary TB, asbestosis, silicosis and lymphoma. It is elevated in about 75% of patients with untreated sarcoid. The value of using serum ACE to monitor disease activity remains unclear.

The lung function tests depend on severity of the disease. The tuberculin test is negative in 80% of patients with sarcoidosis. Treatment with a corticosteroid should be given to patients with ocular sarcoid, hypercalcaemia, severe or persistent erythema nodosum, myocardial and neurological manifestations of sarcoidosis.

In this question the other diagnoses can be ruled out as follows: Langerhans' cell histiocytosis is unlikely as it usually presents in younger patients and nearly all affected individuals have a history of current or previous smoking; he has a negative (grade 0–1) Heaf test, making TB unlikely, because with the degree of change on the CXR one would expect a positive Heaf test (unless the patient was immunosuppressed) and the patient to be more unwell (also one would expect most Irish citizens to have a positive (up to grade 2) Heaf test due to previous BCG vaccination); berylliosis is a possible alternative, but there is no evidence of exposure; small-cell lung cancer is unusual in a young non-smoker.

Common clinical characteristics of sarcoidosis include:

- Skin:
    erythema nodosum – caution, not always on the shins
    lupus pernio – red crusty lesions, often around the nose
    annular lesion
- Polyuria:
    secondary to hypercalciuria/hypercalcaemia (can also cause renal calculi and nephrocalcinosis)
    secondary to central diabetes insipidus
- Cardiac:
    ventricular arrhythmias
    conduction defects
    cardiomyopathy
    congestive cardiac failure
- Neurological:
    involvement of CNS occurs in 2%
    cranial diabetes insipidus
- Ocular:
    anterior uveitis
    conjunctivitis
    retinal lesions
    keratoconjunctivitis sicca and lacrimal gland enlargement
    optic neuritis
- Metabolic:
    hypercalcaemia and hypercalciuria
- Bone and joints:
    arthralgia
    bone cysts

- Others:
  hepatosplenomegaly
  Löfgren's syndrome (acute sarcoidosis) – triad of bihilar
    lymphadenopathy, arthritis and erythema nodosum.

Case 7

1   **A**   Cystic fibrosis

2   **D**   Sweat test

3   **D**   *Pseudomonas aeruginosa*

This boy has cystic fibrosis. He has had recurrent chest infections secondary to bronchiectasis (confirmed by examination findings and the chest X-ray, also note long line inserted via left antecubital fossa), he is small for his age, has nasal polyps and clubbing. He has mildly deranged liver function tests – secondary to obstruction of biliary ductules in the liver. This can eventually lead to cirrhosis. He has glucose in his urine – pancreatic islet cells are destroyed as the pancreas becomes fibrotic.

The most likely cause of this patient's haemoptysis is secondary to bronchiectasis. Patietns with cystic fibrosis may have offensive stools secondary to pancreatic insufficiency.

Goodpasture's syndrome is a cause of haemoptysis but usually occurs in patients over 16.

Kartagener's syndrome causes bronchiectasis and situs inversus.

The diagnosis of cystic fibrosis is made by a sweat test. A sweat sodium concentration over 60 mmol/L is indicative of cystic fibrosis.

By the time patients are in their teenage years, *Pseudomonas aeruginosa* is the commonest organism to colonise the patient. Patients tend to be infected initially with *Staphylococcus aureus*.

Male cystic fibrosis patients are infertile due to failure of the development of the vas deferens and epididymis.

Treatment is with pancreatic supplements, regular antibiotics, strict glucose control, mucolytics/DNAase and regular physiotherapy with postural drainage. Lung transplantation is also a treatment option once there is severe respiratory compromise.

Case 8

1 **D** Pulmonary oedema

2 **A** Wegener's granulomatosis

3 **A** c-ANCA (anti-proteinase 3)

4 **C** Cyclophosphamide and prednisolone

This is a question about pulmonary-renal syndromes. (For a list see below.)
The raised TLCO and the CXR should make one think of pulmonary haemorrhage. This should narrow the diagnosis down to a vasculitis, Goodpasture's syndrome and SLE.

This patient has Wegener's granulomatosis. The clinical diagnosis is made by the triad of upper respiratory tract (nasal polyps and sinusitis), lower respiratory tract and renal involvement. It is a small-vessel vasculitis associated with granulomas.
Microscopic polyangiitis is characterised by a very similar small-vessel vasculitis without granuloma formation and involvement of the upper respiratory tract.
Legionella pneumonia is unlikely as he is afebrile and there is no evidence of foreign travel or exposure. It again does not have a predilection for the upper respiratory tract.

Goodpasture's syndrome can present like this but the upper respiratory tract signs and symptoms are not typical.

Pulmonary oedema is the least likely diagnosis as the JVP is not elevated and the KCO would be reduced.

The diagnosis of Wegener's granulomatosis is suggested by a positive c-ANCA with the presence of an antibody to proteinase 3. The chest X-ray usually shows single or multiple nodules, fixed infiltrates or cavities. Diagnosis is usually confirmed with a biopsy. Treatment is with intravenous cyclophosphamide and prednisolone. Plasmapheresis would be first-line treatment if the disease was primarily renal.

Causes of pulmonary-renal syndromes:

- Systemic diseases:
    Wegener's granulomatosis
    microscopic polyangiitis
    Goodpasture's syndrome
    systemic lupus erythematosus
    polyarteritis nodosum
    Henoch–Schönlein purpura
    Churg–Strauss syndrome (renal involvement less common)

- Primary pulmonary disease:
  Legionella pneumonia and interstitial nephritis
  bacterial pneumonia with renal compromise secondary to sepsis
- Others:
  pulmonary oedema with acute renal failure
  uraemic pneumonitis
  right-sided bacterial endocarditis – may cause pulmonary embolic
    lesions and glomerulonephritis
  iatrogenic glomerulonephritis with ciprofloxacin, eg in patients
    given ciprofloxacin for cystic fibrosis.

Case 9

1   **D**   Churg–Strauss syndrome

2   **B**   p-ANCA positive, anti-MPO antibody-positive
    G   Bronchoscopy and bronchoalveolar lavage

This patient has Churg–Strauss syndrome. The patient has systemic symptoms, asthma, eosinophils greater than 1.5×10^9/L and evidence of vasculitis in two or more non-lung organs (Lanham's criteria):

- Cutaneous vasculitis (see picture)
- Mononeuritis multiplex
- A cardiac history.

The American Criteria of Rheumatology require four out of six of the following to be present for a diagnosis of Churg–Strauss syndrome:

- The presence of asthma
- Eosinophils greater than 10% in the peripheral blood
- Evidence of a neuropathy in a vasculitic pattern, eg mononeuritis multiplex
- Transient pulmonary infiltrates
- A history of sinus disease
- Evidence of intravascular eosinophils on biopsy.

Wegener's and microscopic polyangiitis would show renal involvement. The symptoms preceded the erythromycin, making eosinophilic pneumonia unlikely. Allergic bronchopulmonary aspergillosis usually occurs in asthmatics but would not produce the signs and symptoms of vasculitis as in this patient.

Churg–Strauss syndrome is diagnosed clinically with the aid of a chest X-ray, showing lung infiltrates in 77% of patients. CT gives greater resolution. The peripheral blood eosinophilia is matched by marked eosinophils on bronchoalveolar lavage. p-ANCA anti-myeloperoxidase antibody positive is found in about 70% of cases. A renal biopsy would not be useful as the kidneys are not involved in this patient. Lung biopsy would show necrotising angiitis, granulomas and tissue eosinophilia. Giant cells and fibrinoid necrosis are present.

Case 10

1   **B**   Left upper lobe collapse

2   **C**   Allergic bronchopulmonary aspergillosis

3   **C**   Positive skin test/radioallergosorbent test for *Aspergillus fumigatus*

The chest X-ray shows left upper lobe collapse and shows the 'veil sign'. This patient has allergic bronchopulmonary aspergillosis (ABPA). Pulmonary infiltrates, blood eosinophilia and asthma is usually secondary to Churg–Strauss or allergic bronchopulmonary aspergillosis. This patient does not have the diagnostic criteria for Churg–Strauss syndrome. The patient working as a baker is irrelevant – occupational asthma is unlikely to cause a productive cough or these chest X-ray features.

ABPA is suspected in any patient with asthma who has an abnormal chest X-ray and high peripheral blood eosinophilia (in this case by adding together all the differentials the eosinophil count is > 2). The chest X-ray may show diffuse pulmonary infiltrates, and pulmonary, lobar or segmental collapse occur as transient features. The most common cause is sensitivity to *Aspergillus fumigatus* spores.

The diagnostic criteria include:

- Asthma (in most cases)
- Peripheral eosinophilia of > 0.5 × 10⁹/L
- Abnormal chest X-ray (infiltrates, segmental or lobar collapse)
- Positive skin tests/RAST to an extract of *A. fumigatus*
- *A. fumigatus* IgG serum-precipitating antibodies
- Raised total IgE
- Fungal hyphae of *A. fumigatus* on microscopy of sputum.

The lung and eosinophils:

- Loeffler's syndrome (eosinophils about 10% of blood WCC), also known as acute eosinophilic pneumonia/simple eosinophilic pneumonia. Mild self-limiting illness with transient migratory pulmonary shadows. Associated with parasitic infections, drug allergies and exposure to inorganic chemicals.
- Tropical pulmonary eosinophilia (eosinophils more than 20%) – in tropical countries usually due to migrating larvae of the filarial worms *Wucheria bancrofti* and *Brugia malayi*.

- Chronic/prolonged pulmonary eosinophilia (eosinophils > 20%) – eosinophilic pneumonia persisting for more than 1 month. Chronic debilitating illness characterised by malaise, weight loss, fever and dyspnoea.
- Allergic bronchopulmonary aspergillosis (eosinophils 5–20%) as in this case.
- Churg–Strauss syndrome (eosinophils 5–20%) – see Case 9 – associated with asthma.
- Hypereosinophilic syndrome (eosinophils > 20%) – eosinophilic infiltration of various organs – eg lungs, heart, bone marrow. Can be associated with an eosinophilic arteritis.
- External agents – drugs, toxins, parasitic infection.

Case 11

1   **D**   Mesothelioma

2   **A**   VATS biopsy

The clue is in the question – her husband who has died worked as a plumber. She is a housewife (she has never worked outside the home), so it is assumed she washed her husband's overalls and was therefore exposed to asbestos. She has systemic symptoms as well as a pleural effusion, making the most likely diagnosis malignant mesothelioma.

Video-assisted thoracoscopy surgery is the investigation of choice as it has the highest diagnostic yield. Prophylactic radiotherapy should be given to the operation site.

The chest X-ray shows pleural thickening and an effusion on the right. There is a holly-leaf pleural plaque on the left, consistent with previous asbestos exposure. Incidentally, there is pericardial calcification.

Case 12

1   **B**   *Pneumocystis carinii* pneumonia (PCP)

2   **D**   Indirect immunofluorescence of the bronchoalveolar lavage (BAL)

3   **B**   HIV

4   **E**   Intravenous high-dose co-trimoxazole ± steroids

For the purpose of the exam – people who have lived abroad (especially Africa and South America), businessmen who work abroad, homosexuals and intravenous drug abusers are more likely to have HIV.

This lady has HIV – the history of living in Zimbabwe and the low lymphocyte count are the clues. *Pneumocystis carinii* is the most common opportunistic infection to cause pneumonia in AIDS – especially when the CD4 count is below 200/mm³. It accounts for about 50% of cases of pneumonia in AIDS and 40% of all AIDS-defining illnesses.

Patients usually present with fever, dry cough and breathlessness. They are usually hypoxic and desaturate on exercise.

In PCP the chest X-ray usually shows bilateral interstitial shadowing and cysts in the mid and lower zones. However, the CXR may be normal. Pneumothorax (because the cysts rupture) may be present in up to 10%.

Diagnosis is made by staining induced sputum or BAL with indirect immunofluorescence with monoclonal antibodies. Conventional stains such as silver staining can be used but, currently, immunostaining is the most common technique.

Treatment is with high-flow oxygen and high does co-trimoxazole. Prednisolone should be added in severe cases (PO$_2$ < 9.5 kPa).

Other respiratory diseases associated with immunosuppression, in particular with HIV and AIDS, include:

- Tuberculosis
- Other bacterial pneumonias, including *Mycobacterium avium intracellulare*
- *Cryptococcus* (other fungi include – *Candida, Histoplasma, Nocardia,* and *Aspergillus fumigatus*)
- CMV pneumonitis (other viruses include *herpes simplex*, Epstein–Barr virus)
- Toxoplasmosis
- Kaposi's sarcoma
- Lymphoma.

Case 13

1   **C**   Urinary 5-hydroxyindoleacetic acid
     E   Bronchoscopy and biopsy

2   **C**   Bronchial carcinoid

3   **A**   Surgery

4   **D**   Right upper lobe collapse

This patient has bronchial carcinoid. It commonly presents between the ages of 50 and 70 and is unrelated to smoking. Bronchial carcinoid tumours are the most indolent form of a spectrum of neuroendocrine tumours of the lung that include small-cell cancer as the most malignant. They are thought to arise from Kulchitsky's cells in the bronchial mucosa. They usually secrete serotonin and arise from the large bronchi. Patients may present with a mass, which is usually centrally located (as in this case – CXR shows right upper lobe collapse), or with recurrent chest infections, haemoptysis, chest pain and wheeze. Flushing (which may be precipitated by alcohol, food ingestion, stress or emotion) and diarrhoea may occur. However, patients are commonly asymptomatic and the tumour is found incidentally.

Carcinoid syndrome occurs when there are secondaries in the liver which release serotonin into the systemic circulation. However, symptoms of carcinoid syndrome may rarely occur in bronchial carcinoid in the absence of metastases as the bronchial tree drains straight into the systemic circulation.

Diagnosis is by detection of 5-hydroxyindoleacetic acid (the metabolite of serotonin) in the urine and bronchial carcinoid is usually seen and diagnosed by bronchoscopy and biopsy.

The treatment of choice of bronchial carcinoid is surgical resection. Flushing may be controlled with somatostatin analogues.

Pellagra may occur due to tumour uptake of tryptophan, the precursor of nicotinic acid.

Case 14

1   **D**   Acute mountain sickness

2   **D**   Acetazolamide

3   **E**   High-altitude cerebral oedema

4   **A**   Immediate transfer down the mountain

There are three types of altitude illness. Acute mountain sickness (AMS), high-altitude cerebral oedema (HACE) and high-altitude pulmonary oedema (HAPE). This man has acute mountain sickness. The exact cause is unknown but it is thought to be secondary to cerebral oedema and raised intracranial pressure. It is more common in people who live at low altitude.

Symptoms and signs of AMS are non-specific; however, diagnosis can be made using the criteria named in 'The Lake Louise Score', namely, the setting of recent gain in altitude, the presence of headache and at least one of the following symptoms:

• Gastrointestinal – anorexia, nausea and vomiting
• Fatigue and weakness
• Dizziness or light-headedness
• Difficulty sleeping.

He does not improve and progresses to develop ataxia and drowsiness. This is the development of high-altitude cerebral oedema, which can be considered as end-stage AMS.

Treatment is immediate descent, oxygen and intravenous dexamethasone.

Acetazolamide may be used for prevention and treatment of AMS. It is a carbonic anhydrase inhibitor which causes an intracellular acidosis. It has a diuretic effect which can be useful in AMS/HACE and HAPE. It is also beneficial as it shifts the oxygen-dissociation curve to the right and therefore at lower partial pressures, more oxygen is released to the tissues.

Case 15

1   **E**   Bronchiectasis

2   **C**   High-resolution CT

3   **A**   Kartagener's syndrome

4   **C**   Ciliary electron microscopy

This man has bronchiectasis. Clinical features include recurrent chest infections with the production of copious amounts of mucopurulent sputum. Other symptoms include dyspnoea, wheeze and pleuritic chest pain. Patients are usually clubbed and course crackles are heard in affected areas.

The investigation of choice is a high-resolution CT, demonstrating bronchial dilatation and wall thickening.

The unifying diagnosis is Kartagener's syndrome – sinus inversus, sinusitis and bronchiectasis. The clues are the appendectomy scar in the left iliac fossa and the chest X-ray showing dextracardia. Diagnosis is confirmed with an epithelial (nasal or bronchial) brush or biopsy. These are examined to determine if cilia demonstrate normal co-ordination, beat frequency and beat pattern. Cross-sections of the cilia are also examined by electron microscopy and specific defects of structure visualised, eg absence of dynein arms.

Young's syndrome is bronchiectasis associated with azoospermia and sinusitis in males.

Case 16

1   **B**   Extrinsic allergic alveolitis (EAA)

2   **B**   Avian serum precipitins

This patient has pulmonary fibrosis, demonstrated by the slowly progressive shortness of breath, type I hypoxia and restrictive lung function tests with reduced TLCO and KCO. The chest X-ray shows reticular nodular shadowing. The diagnosis is extrinsic allergic alveolitis secondary to pigeons – bird fancier's lung. This is caused by inhaled avian serum proteins (usually IgA) present in the pigeons' feathers and excreta. It is a hypersensitivity pneumonitis caused by a specific immunological response to inhaled organic dusts. EAA may present either as an acute or a chronic disease. This patient has chronic disease as it has progressed to pulmonary fibrosis.

The diagnosis of extrinsic allergic alveolitis is made by:

- Identifying a potential source of antigen
- Characteristic clinical features – this patient has chronic EAA and presents with similar features to pulmonary fibrosis – clubbing tends to occur later (CFA would typically be associated with clubbing)
- Characteristic radiology (usually upper lobe fibrosis)
- Lung function tests – showing a restrictive defect with reduced carbon monoxide gas transfer
- Demonstrating precipitating antibodies (precipitins) in the patient's serum
- Resolution or improvement of symptoms following avoidance of exposure to the cause.

Treatment is avoidance of the antigen. Corticosteroids improve recovery in acute attacks but do not seem to provide long-term benefit. They are not usually helpful once fibrosis has occurred.

Other causes of EAA include:

- Farmer's lung, due to *Micropolyspora faeni* and *Thermoactinomyces* in mouldy hay, straw and grain
- Bagassosis due to *Thermoactinomyces sacchari* in sugar cane processing
- Malt worker's lung due to *Aspergillus clavatus*
- Mushroom worker's lung due to thermophilic actinomycetes
- Ventilation and water related contamination eg due to thermophilic actinomycetes contaminating air-conditioning systems.
- Veterinary workers and animal handlers
- Workers in milling and construction, eg wood dust pneumonitis due to *alternaria* sp.

Psittacosis is an infection caused by *Chlamydia psittacosis*. It usually presents with a sudden onset of fever, dry cough and headache following a recent exposure to birds.

Causes of upper-zone fibrosis:

- Progressive massive fibrosis/coal worker's pneumoconiosis
- Ankylosing spondylitis
- Sarcoid/silicosis
- Tuberculosis
- Extrinsic allergic alveolitis
- Radiation (depending on site).

Case 17

1 **B** Pulmonary fibrosis

2 **B** Amiodarone

3 **D** Open lung biopsy

This man has pulmonary fibrosis – gradual onset of shortness of breath and dry cough. He is clubbed and has fine inspiratory crackles. Lung function tests are restrictive and he has type I respiratory failure. Chest X-ray shows small lung fields and reticular nodular shadowing.

Next you have to look for a cause. He has a photosensitive rash on his face, atrial fibrillation and abnormal thyroid function, suggesting that he is on amiodarone. Pulmonary fibrosis/alveolitis is an important side effect of long-term amiodarone administration.

Other side effects of amiodarone include:

- Hyper- and hypothyroidism
- Peripheral sensory neuropathy
- Hepatitis
- Photosensitivity
- Ataxia
- Corneal microdeposits (reversible)
- Metallic taste
- Arrhythmias (*torsades de pointes*).

A number of drugs cause pulmonary fibrosis – see below.

Diagnosis is made by a combination of clinical findings, lung function tests, CXR, BAL and high-resolution CT. It is confirmed with an open lung biopsy.

If there was no obvious cause for the pulmonary fibrosis, the answer would be cryptogenic fibrosing alveolitis, also known as 'idiopathic pulmonary fibrosis'.

Drugs causing pulmonary fibrosis:

(For full list see www. Pneumotox.com)

- Antibiotics – nitrofurantoin
- Cardiovascular – amiodarone, β-blockers
- Chemotherapeutic – bleomycin, busulfan, cyclophosphamide, carmustine, lomustine, methotrexate, melphalan, mitomycin C, nitrosureas, sulfasalazine, 5-fluorouracil (5FU)
- Drugs used to treat rheumatoid arthritis – sulfasalazine, penicillamine, cyclophosphamide, methotrexate, gold
- Drugs used to treat migraine – ergotamine, ergots, methysergide
- Others:
  bromocriptine
  radiation
  dothiepin
  pesticides
  high-flow oxygen.

Causes of lower-zone fibrosis:

- Drugs
- Connective tissue disease
- Asbestosis
- Idiopathic pulmonary fibrosis

Case 18

1   **C**   Primary pneumothorax

2   **D**   Lateral decubitus chest X-ray

3   **A**   Analgesia and discharge with follow-up in the clinic

A synchronous click with the heart sounds is a recognised sign of a small left apical pneumothorax. He is a tall thin man and a smoker, which are both risk factors for developing a pneumothorax. There is a strong association between pneumothoraces and smoking. The most recent British Thoracic Society (BTS) guidelines[1,2] suggest that if the postero-anterior (PA) chest X-ray is normal and a small pneumothorax is suspected, a lateral decubitus chest X-ray provides added information in up to 14% of cases. Expiratory films add little and are not recommended. The treatment of a primary pneumothorax with a rim of air of < 2 cm is to discharge and follow up as an outpatient. Patients should be given analgesia if required and clear instructions to return if their symptoms get any worse.

[1] http://www.brit-thoracic.org.uk/
[2] Pleural Disease Group, Standards of Care Committee. 2003. BTS Guidelines on Pleural Disease. *Thorax*, 58 (Suppl 2).

Case 19

1   **B**   Insertion of an intercostal drain

2   **C**   Refer to thoracic surgeons

This man has a secondary pneumothorax as he has underlying lung disease. The management is different for primary (no underlying pulmonary disease) and secondary (underlying pulmonary disease) pneumothoraces. Current guidelines[1] suggest that an intercostal drain should be inserted if the patient is breathless, over 50 years old and there is a rim of air of > 2 cm from the chest wall on a standard size chest X-ray. This patient fits all the above criteria.

Suction should not be applied immediately. It should be applied after 48 hours if the lung is not fully re-expanded or if there is a persistent air leak. Suction should be low-pressure (−10 to −20 cmH$_2$O), high-volume.

Because this patient has a persistent air leak despite suction, they should be referred to the thoracic surgeons. The exact timing of referral remains contentious. For secondary pneumothoraces, an early thoracic surgical referral is recommended.

[1] http:www.brit-thoracic.org.uk
'Introduction to the Methods Used in the Generation of the British Thoracic Society Guidelines for the Management of Pleural Diseases', 2003. *Thorax*: 58 (Suppl. 2).

Case 20

1   **B**   Add an inhaled long-acting β$_2$-agonist

2   **A**   High-flow oxygen, oral/intravenous steroids, salbutamol and ipratropium bromide nebuliser

3   **C**   Refer to ICU for intubation

This woman is on step 2 of the asthma treatment ladder – she is on a low/moderate dose inhaled steroids (800 mg/day). A trial of an alternative agent should be added prior to increasing inhaled steroids. The first choice of additional therapy would be a long-acting β$_2$-agonist as this improves lung function and symptoms and decreases exacerbations. If this did not improve her symptoms, she should stop the long-acting β$_2$-agonist and try a leukotriene receptor antagonist or theophylline.

After stopping her inhalers she is no longer on any medication to control her asthma. She presents to A&E with symptoms and signs of a severe asthma exacerbation – inability to complete a sentence in one breath, respiratory rate > 25/min, tachycardia > 110 bpm and PEFR < 50%. The correct management is high-flow oxygen as patients with pure asthma do not retain carbon dioxide; salbutamol and ipratropium bromide nebulisers driven by oxygen; steroid therapy – prednisolone 40 mg orally if the patient is able to take oral medication, or 100 mg intravenous hydrocortisone. Intravenous magnesium should be given in life-threatening asthma or if there is no response to initial therapy. Intravenous aminophylline can also be used. The best answer is therefore 'A'.

The patient deteriorates and develops signs of life-threatening asthma – a silent chest, a PCO_2 > 6 kPa and a fall in pH. Others signs of life-threatening asthma include: confusion, exhaustion or coma, bradycardia, hypotension, PEFR < 30% predicted or best, severe hypoxaemia (PaO_2 < 8 kPa) despite oxygen therapy. This patient now needs intubation and transfer to ICU. Non-invasive ventilation is not used in asthma at present and it is unlikely to ever replace intubation in life-threatening asthma.[1]

[1] http://www.brit-thoracic.org.uk
'The BTS/SIGN British Guideline on the Management of Asthma', 2003. *Thorax*: 58 (Suppl. 1).

Case 21

1   **C**   Thoracoplasty

2   **D**   Tuberculosis

This lady had tuberculosis in the 1940s, prior to the use of antituberculosis chemotherapy. She had a thoracoplasty, which was one of the main surgical treatments for tuberculosis between 1930 and 1955. Several ribs were resected, which reduced the thoracic volume and collapsed the underlying lung. The aim was to close the tuberculous cavity and 'rest the lung'. Control of pulmonary tuberculosis and survival was good. However, patients were left with severe chest deformity and the associated respiratory compromise, a restrictive defect.

Case 22

1 **D** Acute on chronic respiratory acidosis

2 **E** Reduce inspired oxygen concentration to 28% and repeat arterial blood gases

3 **A** Obstructive airways disease

This patient has an acute on chronic respiratory acidosis. The high bicarbonate and base excess shows that there is an underlying chronic respiratory acidosis with renal compensation. The acidosis and high CO_2 indicate an acute respiratory acidosis. If this was acute without a chronic element then, for a PCO_2 of 10.91 one would expect the pH to be lower.

This question is about oxygen therapy in COPD. The diagnosis of COPD is suggested from the CXR and flow-volume curve, which shows the classic shape for COPD. In some patients with COPD, respiratory drive depends on their degree of hypoxia rather than the usual dependence on hypercapnia. Although it is important to prevent life-threatening hypoxia, uncontrolled oxygen therapy should be used with caution. This patient has a suppressed respiratory drive and carbon dioxide narcosis secondary to high-flow oxygen. He was able to tell the ambulance crew that he had no chest pain at home; he was then given high-flow oxygen and his GCS dropped. Note on arrival at A&E he scored 2/5 for verbal response and therefore would not be able to give any information. The immediate management is therefore to reduce the inspired oxygen concentration and repeat the arterial blood gases. If by doing this the patient becomes hypoxic or remains acidotic, they should then be referred for non-invasive ventilation.[1]

[1] National Collaborating Centre for Chronic Conditions. 2004. Chronic obstructive pulmonary disease. National clinical guideline on management of chronic obstructive pulmonary disease in adults in primary and secondary care. *Thorax*, 59 (Suppl 1), 1–232.

Case 23

1 **B** Left lower lobe collapse

2 **E** CT chest/upper abdomen and bronchoscopy

3 **C** Small-cell carcinoma of the lung

4 **D** Chemotherapy

5 **B** 2.74 mmol/L

The chest X-ray shows left lower lobe collapse. There is loss of volume of the left hemithorax and the classical sail sign behind the heart.

This man has a lung malignancy – weight loss, haemoptysis, dyspnoea and hypercalcaemia. The aim of this question is to ensure you know the paraneoplastic syndromes associated with certain types of lung cancer. The clues are the:

- Hyponatraemia secondary to the syndrome of inappropriate antidiuretic hormone secretion
- The proximal weakness and hyporeflexia, which, along with autonomic features, represents Lambert–Eaton myasthenic syndrome.

These are seen more frequently with small-cell lung cancer. Ectopic ACTH production is also associated but rare.

Squamous-cell carcinoma is associated with:

- Gynaecomastia
- Hyperthyroidism
- Hypertropic pulmonary osteoarthropathy (HPOA) – finger clubbing, periostitis and arthritis
- Hypercalcaemia – usually secondary to bone metastases but rarely may be secondary to secretion of PTH-related peptide.

Common to both:

- Hypercalcaemia – the corrected calcium here is 2.74 mmol/L – due to bony metastases. If albumin is < 40 g/L, corrected calcium = $[Ca^{2+}] + 0.02 \times \{40 - [alb]\}$ mmol/L
- Clubbing
- Smoking – he is likely to be a smoker or ex-smoker and have COPD as he is on inhalers.

A histological diagnosis is important, as is accurate staging. Therefore the most appropriate next investigation would be a bronchoscopy and biopsy and a staging CT scan. Following this, a bone scan would be useful to confirm bone metastases. Since this patient has deranged liver function tests and hypercalcaemia it is likely he has metastatic disease. Treatment of small-cell lung cancer is primarily chemotherapy as metastases tend to occur early. Surgical resection may be considered in combination with chemotherapy if it presented as a solitary pulmonary nodule. Palliative care involvement is important for symptomatic control or if the patient is unsuitable for other treatment options.

Case 24

1 **A** Fixed extrathoracic airflow obstruction

2 **E** Goitre

The flow–volume loop shows a fixed extrathoracic airflow obstruction – both inspiratory and expiratory flow is blunted. This is caused by the large goitre shown on the chest X-ray. In extrathoracic obstructions flow tends to be constant throughout the first part of expiration rather than decelerating. The inspiratory flow is even more reduced. Normally, inspiratory flow is promoted by the negative intrathoracic pressure pulling the intrathoracic airways open. The extrathoracic obstruction prevents this from happening, thus reducing inspiratory flow. Another cause of fixed extrathoracic obstruction is tracheal stenosis. Variable extrathoracic obstruction does not affect the expiratory flow. Causes include: tracheal tumours, vocal cord paralysis and pharyngeal muscle weakness.

Case 25

1   **C**   Serum α_1-antitrypsin

2   **E** α_1-Antitrypsin deficiency

Alpha$_1$-antitrypsin deficiency is a rare autosomal recessive disease associated with the development of premature panlobular emphysema. Patients usually present with progressive increasing shortness of breath and weight loss. Cor pulmonale and polycythaemia occur later in the course of the disease. A chest X-ray usually shows bilateral bibasal emphysema. Lung function tests show an obstructive picture and the RV:TLC ratio is raised, indicating gas trapping. There are a number of different phenotypes depending on the serum level of α_1-antitrypsin:
Pi – protease inhibitor
M – normal allele
S, Z and null are disease alleles

Phenotype	α_1-Antitrypsin level	Disease
PiMM	Normal	
PiMS	80%	
PiMZ	60%	
PiSS	60%	
PiSZ	40%	
PiZZ	10–15%	Liver cirrhosis/premature emphysema
Pi Null Null	nil	Premature emphysema

Treatment is similar to that of asthma. Alpha$_1$-antitrypsin replacement can be given weekly or monthly and is recommended for those with very low serum levels and abnormal lung function. Patients should be encouraged to stop smoking.

Case 26

1   **C**   Epworth score
    H   Sleep studies

2   **C**   Advise to lose weight

3   **B**   Alcohol excess

This patient has obstructive sleep apnoea (OSA) – insomnia, daytime somnolence, morning headache and obesity. Other symptoms include poor concentration during the day and partners may describe snoring followed by apnoeic episodes. Diagnosis is made using the Epworth score – which is a measure of daytime somnolence – and sleep studies, which would show apnoeic/hypopnoeic episodes associated with desaturations, increase in heart rate and arousal from sleep. Although treatment is with nocturnal non-invasive ventilation (NIV), initially management should be to advise weight loss as this may improve his symptoms and thus prevent the need for NIV. Early morning headaches can be caused by a hypercapnia. Therefore if a patient has hypercapnia and were referred for non-invasive ventilation, bilevel positive airway pressure (eg BiPAP) would be better than CPAP (continuous positive airway pressure).

It is important to exclude underlying causes – this patient has a history of gout which, together with the raised MCV and low platelets, suggests alcohol consumption, which can precipitate the problem. Hypothyroidism, acromegaly and sedating drugs also need to be excluded. Retrognathia can cause OSA and large tonsils may obstruct the airway.

Case 27

1   **B**   Yellow-nail syndrome

This girl has yellow-nail syndrome which is a rare condition consisting of the triad of primary lymphoedema, recurrent pleural effusions and dystrophic yellow nails. It is associated with bronchiectasis and sinusitis. Pleural fluid is typically a clear exudate in which lymphocytes predominate. The underlying abnormality is hypoplasia of the lymphatics with impaired drainage. This results in subungual oedema, lymphoedema and pleural effusions.

Meigs' syndrome is a rare syndrome with an association between pleural effusions, ascites and benign ovarian tumours – usually fibromas.

Filariasis is one of the most common causes of lymphoedema secondary to microfilariae being introduced into the skin by mosquitoes and migrating to the lymphatics. It can be associated with chylous pleural effusions.

Case 28

1   **A**   Oesophageal rupture

Oesophageal rupture is a serious condition following trauma, violent vomiting, endoscopic procedures or associated with malignancy. Spillage of gastric contents into the pleura causes shock and pain. The chest X-ray usually shows a left pleural effusion or hydropneumothorax. There may also be air in the soft tissues (as in this patient). Pleural fluid is an exudate and amylase levels are high. The ratio of pleural fluid amylase to serum amylase is > 1.0. Iso-enzyme analysis can be useful as oesophageal rupture will show the amylase to be salivary in origin.

Diagnosis is made radiologically using water-soluble contrast. Surgical treatment is required and mortality is high.

Case 29

1   **B**   Occupational asthma

This man has occupational asthma secondary to isocyanates which are found in spray paints used to spray cars. Occupational asthma is characterised by airway obstruction and/or bronchial hyper-reactivity induced by a person's occupation. His spirometry reveals an obstructive picture with a hyper-responsive histamine challenge test.

Other occupations commonly associated with occupational asthma that may come up in the MRCP exam include: bakers, vets, hairdressers, pharmaceutical workers, welders, roofers and textile workers.

Case 30

1   **B**   CMV pneumonitis

2   **A**   Intravenous ganciclovir

This patient has a cytomegalovirus (CMV) infection. CMV is one of the most frequent opportunistic infections in patients with advanced HIV disease. A CD4 count below 50 cells/mm³ carries a high risk of the disease. It can cause hepatitis, colitis, retinitis, pneumonitis, radiculopathy and encephalitis. Clinically and radiologically, CMV pneumonia mimics *Pneumocystis carinii* pneumonia (PCP). However, this patient was on prophylactic co-trimoxazole, making PCP less likely. The reduced visual acuity and abnormal liver function tests also are more in keeping with CMV. In the immunosuppressed, serology may be of little value. Diagnosis is made by polymerase chain reaction (PCR) of serum. Histological staining of transbronchial biopsies may demonstrate the pathognomonic 'owl's eye' cells. Other techniques include rapid culture methods such as DEAFF (detection of early antigen fluorescent foci) by monoclonal antibody.

Treatment is with intravenous ganciclovir.

Case 31

1   **D**   X-linked hypogammaglobulinaemia

2   **B**   Measure immunoglobulins

This patient has X-linked hypogammaglobulinaemia. The main clue is the low total protein with a normal albumin, demonstrating low levels of globulins. Patients usually present in childhood with recurrent infections, which result in bronchiectasis if untreated, and malabsorption, in a similar way to patients with cystic fibrosis. All immunoglobulin classes and B cells and plasma cells are reduced. The defect is in the differentiation of pre-B cells into B cells. T cells are normal. The gene defect is on the long arm of the X chromosome, making it an X-linked condition.

Treatment is with intravenous immunoglobulin therapy which, if started early, can prevent progression of disease.

The chest X-ray shows bronchiectasis – parallel thickened bronchial walls with a 'tram track' appearance.

Case 32

1   **D**   Echocardiogram

2   **C**   Bilateral diaphragmatic weakness

In bilateral diaphragmatic weakness, patients commonly present with breathlessness on exertion and when lying flat. It can be associated with sleep apnoea, resulting in daytime somnolence and headaches. The symptoms are due to the paroxysmal movement of the diaphragm during inspiration. In the supine position, expansion of the ribs results in movement of abdominal contents into the chest, aided by gravity. Symptoms can be worse when standing up to the waist in water as this counteracts the effects of gravity and prevents outward movement of the abdomen during inspiration and therefore produces a similar situation to being in the supine position.

A chest X-ray may show relatively small lung fields and basal linear shadowing due to subsegmental collapse. A SNIF test (diaphragmatic screening on ultrasound) will show paradoxical movement of the diaphragm, particularly on sniffing. Blood gases may show a type II respiratory failure, particularly at night. Lung function tests classically show a low vital capacity, which falls further in the supine position. All lung volumes except the residual volume are reduced. The gas transfer tends to mildly impaired with a normal KCO.

Treatment is with non-invasive ventilation.

The numbers in this index refer to the chapter and question numbers. The topics shown may not always be in the question, but may appear in the explanatory answers.

PasTest

PasTest has been established since 1972 and is the leading provider of exam-related medical revision courses and books in the UK. The company has a dedicated customer services team to ensure that doctors can easily get up-to-date information about our products and to ensure that their orders are dealt with efficiently. Our extensive experience means that we are always one step ahead when it comes to knowledge of the current trends and contents of the Royal College exams.

PasTest revision books have helped thousands of candidates prepare for their exams. These may be purchased through bookshops, over the telephone or online at our website. All books are reviewed prior to publication to ensure that they mirror the needs of candidates and therefore act as an invaluable aid to exam preparation.

100% Money Back Guarantee
We're sure you will find our study books invaluable, but in the unlikely event that you are not entirely happy, we will give you your money back – guaranteed.

Delivery to your Door
With a busy lifestyle, nobody enjoys walking to the shops for something that may or may not be in stock. Let us take the hassle and deliver direct to your door. We will despatch your book within 24 hours of receiving your order. We also offer free delivery on books for medical students to UK addresses.

How to Order
www.pastest.co.uk
To order books safely and securely online, shop at our website.

Telephone: +44 (0)1565 752000
Have your credit card to hand when you call.
Fax: +44 (0) 1565 650264
Fax your order with your debit or credit card details.

PasTest Ltd, FREEPOST, Knutsford, Cheshire WA16 7BR
Send your order with your cheque (made payable to PasTest Ltd) and debit or credit card details to the above address. (Please complete your address details on the reverse of the cheque.)